Acknowledgements

This book was made possible by the vision of Michel Boileau, MD and Gary Hoffman, MD. These two men shared a passion and a commitment to provide information and products supporting good pelvic floor health for women, recognizing the silence and privacy that go along with this health issue. A special thanks goes to Michael S. Wax, President and CEO of DesChutes Medical Products, Inc. for his support of this project. I am grateful to Diane Larson, PhD, RN Judy Hoffman, Lisa Buan Hammermann, Kathie Sharp, Shelly Makleff, Denise Bestwick, Larry Katz and Douglas Johnson, MD for their review and comments. I am especially indebted to Brandi Gilmore for structuring the type, creating the illustrations, and seeing the project through from beginning to end with personal enthusiasm.

My most sincere thanks is reserved for Charlene, Sara, Frankie, Marge, Carolyn, Stella and all of the other women who have taught me the devastating impact that bladder leakage or pelvic floor relaxation can have on quality of life. I have known the rewards of having helped many of them. I hope this book can reach even more women with the lessons they have shared.

This book is now for you, the reader, with the hope that you can find solutions to relieve symptoms of incontinence and improve your quality of life. I welcome your comments at dsmith@deschutesmed.com.

Dorothy B. Smith, RN,MS,CWOCN,FAAN

Bladder Control is No Accident™
A Woman's Guide

Special sections on:
Exercise incontinence
Incontinence during intercourse
Pregnancy
Menopause
Nocturia
Bedwetting in children

Dorothy B. Smith
RN, MS, CWOCN, FAAN

DesChutes Medical Products, Inc.
Bend, Oregon

Published by
DesChutes Medical Products, Inc.
1011 SW Emkay Drive, Suite 104
Bend, OR 97702
DMP Press is a unit of DesChutes Medical Products, Inc.
Call 1-800-323-1363 for additional copies

ISBN: 0-9708686-0-X

This book is not intended to be used in place of medical
evaluation, diagnosis or treatment.

Cover design and illustrations by Brandi Gilmore

Visit our website http://www.deschutesmed.com

Printed in the United States of America by
Maverick Publications
Bend, Oregon

Dedication

Dedicated to Michel A. Boileau, M.D.

I met a young Dr. Boileau when he was a fellow in urologic cancer at The University of Texas M.D. Anderson Cancer Center in Houston, Texas. Dr. Boileau impressed me early on with his caring nature, intelligence and inventive mind. But when he made home visits to a dying prostate patient—who lived 300 miles away in another state, I was touched. Twenty years later, he continues to be a patient advocate for quality of life. Incontinence is not a field that physicians fight over. Few are even interested in the challenge of helping patients with this problem. Dr. Boileau is one of those who is. He is continually making efforts to provide avenues of care where the patient can be an active partner in her care. His support and review of this self-help guide is but one of his many efforts.

~DBS

Foreword

We learn very early in life that it is not acceptable to wet ourselves. Children are often ostracized if they are not "Toilet Trained" within the early preschool years. It is not surprising that adults who become incontinent feel the need to hide this distressing symptom and sometimes limit most social activities. It was so embarrassing that one didn't even discuss it with a physician. Most men and women felt they were alone with this problem until the past few years when advertisements began appearing on television and in magazines selling products for "adults who wet".

It was my good fortune to learn the importance of exercising the supporting pelvic muscles in the 1950's when my physician husband trained under Dr. Kegel. As a Nurse and Lamaze teacher I spent many years encouraging women to make the "Kegel" exercise a part of their daily routine. Years after I learned, with great personal disappointment, that exercising these muscles did not necessarily prevent urine leakage later in life.

It has now become evident that many younger women as well as men have both leakage and urge incontinence. Often these are people who are extremely healthy and active. Stress from sports, childbirth, surgery, certain occupations and other causes can create a situation that may not be permanently eliminated even with bladder surgery.

Dot Smith has written a very comprehensive self-help manual providing a way to understand both the causes of incontinence and methods for improving bladder control. While other books have been available, this is the first one that is easy to follow and includes the very latest in bladder training feedback methods.

As a psychologist I often have to teach behavioral methods for change. This can be tiresome and difficult unless one has good guidance and support. I feel that this manual provides both. I encourage all medical and health professionals to read about this condition and encourage your patients/clients to discuss any such difficulties so their overall health and social life can be enhanced. Dot Smith has provided us all a wonderful resource.

Diane Larson, Ph.D., R.N.
Los Gatos, CA

Table of Contents

The Doctor Speaks

After twenty years as a practicing urologist I have concluded that urinary incontinence may be the most troubling problem that brings patients to me. The statistics on incontinence are staggering, in that more than 25 million people are afflicted, and most are too embarrassed to even mention it to their doctors. So it remains undiagnosed and untreated.

The social costs are very high because of this. Social isolation, depression, infections, hospitalizations are just a few of the consequences. In fact, the single most common problem that compels a family to put an elder in a nursing home is urinary incontinence.

It is troubling to note the incredible growth in the adult diaper business since June Allison was brave enough to become a spokesperson for adult incontinence. The dollar sales for adult diapers are now in the billions, and most of the feminine hygiene pads are actually sold to contain urine leakage. Most people believe that incontinence is either a natural consequence of aging and is untreatable, or is only treatable with surgery or expensive medicines. So they simply buy diapers or pads and endure the discomfort, the skin breakdown, the infections, the odor and the embarrassment.

Dorothy Smith's book is long overdue. Ms. Smith is a highly

regarded specialist in the treatment of urinary incontinence, and has years of experience helping these patients. Despite the fact that this problem is underdiagnosed and undertreated it is a very treatable problem. Most individuals who are incontinent, up to 80% can be cured or successfully treated without surgery and without medication! The path to continence is often simple and relatively easy. In cases where surgery or medication is required those treatments can be very successful. The fact is that help is available, and most people can be dry.

Bladder Control is No Accident   A Woman's Guide brings to stricken patients or their families the guidance and information necessary to find help and effectively treat urinary incontinence. Ms. Smith explains the different types of incontinence in clear, non-medical terms. This book allows people to privately assess their situations, and show them ways to self treat simple problems, or seek necessary medical treatment for more serious conditions. It provides a private way to gain the confidence of knowledge about incontinence, and overcome the embarrassment and isolation that lead to so much unnecessary suffering. As I said, this book is long overdue.

Michel A. Boileau, M.D., F.A.C.S.
Clinical Professor of Urology
Oregon Health Sciences University

Introduction

Welcome to *Bladder Control is No Accident A Woman's Guide*, your self-help guide to bladder control. As a nurse, I have been clinically involved with patients having urinary and gynecological problems for many years. I have written this book as a self-help guide for women who are eager to improve their bladder control. Although I chose to be academic at times to give knowledge to the reader, I have also inserted some of my professional experiences to give the reader a lighter and more personal view. In some instances I have used words such as "bladder irritant or stimulant" even though the mechanism of how this happens is not known. But these are terms frequently used in lay-persons urinary continence newsletters and "bladder control talk", so I have taken the liberty of using them here. I hope you will find the content and suggestions helpful in reducing your bladder control symptoms and improving your quality of life. Acknowledging the problem, gaining knowledge, and committing to action are the first steps to successfully addressing bladder control issues.

Dorothy B. Smith, RN, MS, FAAN
DesChutes Medical Products, Inc.
Bend, OR

ஐ *Chapter 1* ଓ

Incontinence:
The Silent Companion

Incontinence: The Silent Companion

Is This You?

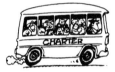

Did you miss the church choir trip
because the church bus did not have toilet?

Do you know every service station or fast
food stop between home and work?

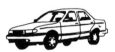

Do you ever feel anxiety when riding in a car with a driver who may
not be considerate about bathroom stops?

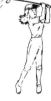

Have you stopped at every rest stop on the golf course
as well as behind a few of the trees?

Does the "fasten your seatbelt"
sign on the airplane make
you immediately need to use the toilet?

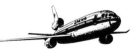

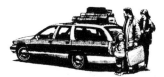
Do you deliberately stop drinking fluids so you won't
leak so much?

Are you insecure about exercising with a
group for fear of leaking urine?

Have you ever considered not taking your diuretic
medication (fluid pill) because you lose control of
your urine after taking it?

Do you view coffee as a "bladder enemy"?

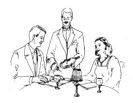
Do you hesitate to stay overnight with a
friend or family?

Have you recently had to go home and
change your clothing after an accident?

Is your personal motto
"never pass up a restroom?"

Does going to the
bathroom frequently
interfere with your
work?

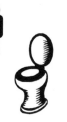

Have you looked for
a bathroom minutes
after just going to one?

Do you get up to go to the bathroom
more than once every night— sometimes not getting
there before having an accident?

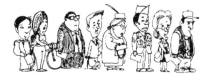

Are you the first in line at the at
the restroom after the movie?
Church? School play?

Do you use a "panty liner" product even
though you are not having your period?

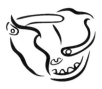

Have you ever been embarrassed because
you leaked urine during sexual activity?

Do you have to plan for "paper products"
as well as groceries in your monthly budget?

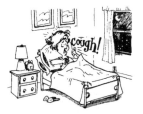

Do you leak urine when you stand up?
Laugh? Cough? Sneeze? Lift? Push?

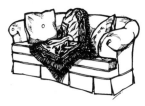

Do you worry about sitting
on the furniture at a friend's house?

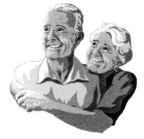

Have you ever thought (or been told)
that leaking urine was a normal
consequence of aging and you would
have to accept it?

The Impact of Incontinence

If you have responded "yes" to any of those situations, you are definitely in a crowd of many women who have had the same or similar experiences. Perhaps there was a laugh or a chuckle when you read some of them. But, in reality, it is not a laughing matter. Urinary incontinence is also known as loss of bladder control, bladder control problems, urinary leakage, or an "accident". Whatever term is used, it essentially is the uncontrollable loss of urine. It is a silent companion to an unknown number of women of all ages. As one patient replied "we go underground with our problem." Reportedly, it affects approximately 20 million women in America. However, it is not easy to get an accurate number of those with incontinence because much of the time urinary leakage remains unreported. Many women, thinking there is no help available, simply tolerate it without asking for help. To a great extent, it is guarded by silence. Only an estimated one in 4 adults with bladder control problems seek professional help or tell a health provider about the problem.

Even though urinary incontinence is mentioned historically in medical texts, it has not received a great deal of attention in the past. Dr. J.L. Newman gives a somewhat cynical perspective to this lack of attention. Writing in a 1962 British Medical Journal article, Old Folk in Wet Beds,[1] Dr. Newman noted that if the wet spot in the bed was blood and not urine, it would get immediate attention. This is true. The presence of blood seems to initiate some type of action. Loss of bladder control is not seen as life threatening, however life altering it may be. Many healthcare professionals dismiss it as being due to old age, a nursing problem, or as something that a "diaper" can fix. However, beyond the inconvenience of being wet, there can be serious consequences of urinary leakage. The following facts are known about a woman with urinary incontinence.

The woman with urinary incontinence:

- is more at risk for **falls** while hurrying to the toilet trying to prevent an "accident"
- is more at risk for urinary tract **infections** and the associated complications

- is more at risk for **skin** breakdown if urine remains on the skin in a pad or clothing
- is more likely to be admitted to a **long-term care** facility when other health problems exist
- has **longer hospital** stays and more frequent admissions
- has to deal with the financial **costs** of buying pads and/or supplies
- has to live with the inconvenience and **embarrassment** of "accidents" in public
- is more likely to be constantly concerned about the location of toilets, even to the point of **restricting** travel or other activities

These consequences are documented by studies in the medical literature. They point out the seriousness of incontinence beyond quality of life issues. Wagner and Hu[2] estimated the annual cost to a person over the age of 65 with incontinence to be $3,565. That is quite a dollar amount for a generation where many are on a fixed income. There are social and psychological consequences of incontinence as well as the physical and economic costs. According to Frost & Sullivan, incontinence supplies rank #1 at $2,210 billion in 2001 projected revenues for medical products. That is just the supplies and does not include the indirect costs related to incontinence. (Medical Device & Diagnostic Industry Dec 2000, 47-56) Incontinence can contribute to inactivity, withdrawal, social isolation, and even depression. Urinary leakage is not a sometime symptom like a headache that occurs occasionally and goes away. It has the potential of being, and frequently is, a several-times-a-day symptom. This can be very challenging to tolerate and frustrating to treat. Dr. Rodney Appell, a urologist formerly at the renowned Cleveland Clinic Foundation in Cleveland, Ohio, and now at Baylor College of Medicine, writes that urinary incontinence "impacts the quality of life more adversely than hypertension, diabetes, and just about any other medical condition except perhaps clinical depression".[3] If you are dealing with incontinence, you personally know the cost, the quality of life issues, the inconvenience, the embarrassment, and the pain of this silent companion. This book offers help for you.

Someone Take Notice!

The 1995 societal cost of incontinence to individuals aged 65 and over was $26.3 billion.[2] That's "B" as in billion; billion dollars! Aside from the quality of life issue that 25 million Americans suffer with incontinence, one would think that something costing this much would have more public attention! More medical attention! More articles at the newsstand! More coverage in the self-help section of the bookstore! A talk show topic! One would think that this problem would have moved out of the silent corner of life! The June Allison television commercials (Depends®, a garment for urinary leakage) and now the Detrol® (medication for overactive bladder) ads are available to the public, but with very specific product marketing. This is certainly a start toward public awareness, but diapers and medications are not the only solutions for this problem. I do not wish bladder control symptoms on anyone, but it would increase public awareness if a person with a recognizable name would say "I had this problem, and this is what I did to solve it". A senator, a sports figure, a music performer, or an actress advocating as a spokesperson for this problem would be a big contribution toward education and public awareness. It would be similar to the Ronald Reagan effect on Alzheimer's Disease, the Bob Dole effect on erectile dysfunction or the Michael J. Fox effect on Parkinson's Disease. Perhaps this attention would help remove some of the hush-hush surrounding the issue of urinary incontinence. How many senators have the opportunity to represent 25 million Americans in their public life? What an opportunity!

"Congressman? Oprah? Paul Harvey? Where are you?"

Now, do you feel better, knowing that you are not the only one dealing with this problem? Or, are you totally depressed, realizing that the problem is so widespread? Without the intent of depressing you further, but to make you more aware of the scope of urinary incontinence, realize that your closest neighbor may be having a similar problem. Those young, fit, super athletes on television or at your

local stadium or high school are not exempt from symptoms of bladder control. Neither is your congresswoman, your pharmacist, your physician, your mother, your sister, your daughter. Having bladder control problems should not cause shame and embarrassment: it is **not** your fault, it is **not** normal, and there **are** treatment options available.

> *Having bladder control problems should not cause shame and embarrassment: it is not your fault, it is not normal, and there are treatment options available.*

Who Has This Problem?

Who, besides you, has his problem??? Here are some real-life examples.

*A*nn

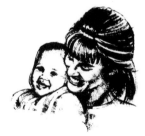

Ann is a 34-year-old homemaker and mother of three young children. Her youngest child is 9 months old. After the birth of her first two children she had a small amount of urinary leakage when she coughed, laughed or sneezed. This lasted only a few weeks and she attributed it to a normal part of having a child. After the birth of her third child, the same problem occurred, but this time it was worse and did not resolve in a few weeks. Ann leaked urine when she laughed, coughed, picked up her infant and even when she had sexual intercourse with her husband. She was very embarrassed and did not know how to deal with her problem or where to turn for help. She started

wearing some menstrual pads that she had on hand, but they were not adequate to keep the urine from spilling on to her clothing. Her doctor never asked about such a problem and she was too embarrassed to bring it up. She thought that it was something she would have to live with forever.

*M*ary

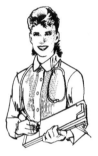

Mary is a 53-year-old mother of three and a nurse. She has Type II diabetes controlled by diet. She leaked urine approximately six times a day. Her "accidents" came when she laughed, coughed, sneezed or exercised. While jogging she had to wear pads to protect her clothing. Even though Mary was a nurse she had not sought medical help for her problem. She said, "I know all of the doctors here. It is too embarrassing."

*A*ngie

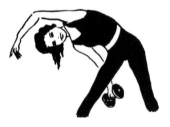

Angie is a 23-year-old competitive swimmer. She is single and very athletic, working out with weights in the gym, swimming, and jogging. For several years she has experienced urinary frequency and sometimes leaked urine while lifting weights or doing sit-ups. She began going to the bathroom more frequently to avoid having accidents. Eventually she was getting up at night 4 to 5 times to go to the bathroom and looking for a rest room every hour or so during the day. She even cut back on her fluid intake during exercise (self-dehydration) to try and reduce her urinary frequency and possible leaks.

Aunt Doris

Doris is a 76-year-old mother of 5 who lives in an assisted living facility near her son. For many years she has experienced loss of bladder control when she laughs, sneezes, or coughs. She learned to deal with this by using tissue or an occasional pad in her panties. She never mentioned this to her healthcare

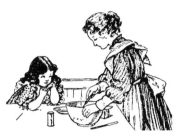

providers or family because she was so embarrassed. The problem began getting worse as she got older. She now has Parkinson's disease and has difficulty getting up and starting to move. She finds that frequently she knows when she needs to go to the bathroom, but cannot get up and get there in time. She is very distressed about her loss of bladder control, the associated odor, and her inability to deal with the leakage. She limits her trips out with her family or with her friends in the facility. She is also fearful that the assisted living home will not let her continue to stay if she cannot regain control of her bladder.

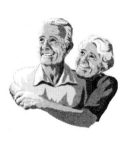

John and Ollie

John, age 83, and his 80-year-old wife, Ollie, live in a retirement village. Both are quite healthy and enjoy moderate activities. For several years, Ollie has experienced a problem with incontinence that is worse at night. She has been to several physicians and tried medications. The medications made her dizzy causing her to fall and break her hip, so they were discontinued. Now John sets his alarm at midnight to help Ollie to the bathroom-and yet sometimes she still leaks, wetting her clothing and the bed. They have not had a full night's rest in months. John buys incontinence pads for Ollie at the grocery store, but they do not keep the bed or her clothing dry. The smell of urine greets them every morning.

*R*andy

Randy is a seven-year-old second grader. He wets his bed almost every night. It is rare for him to get through the night without wetting his bed. He is shy and retiring and does not want to be involved in cub scouts or camping. He loves baseball and would like to play, but is afraid there might be overnight trips involved at the end of season. His father was a bedwetter as a child and eventually outgrew his symptoms. His mother and father are very supportive and do not punish him, but his older brother teases him. His mother has made Randy's pediatrician aware of the problem now and wants to seek help from a specialist. She is afraid Randy's self-esteem and personality are being affected.

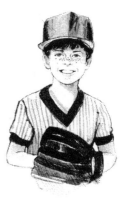

These are stories about real people who have encountered incontinence. Some of their symptoms may sound familiar to you from your own experiences or from those of a family member or friend. However, these people did not remain silent. They all eventually sought help and received successful treatment. Loss of bladder control has long been associated with shame and embarrassment. Today, the shame is not in being wet. The shame is in not receiving appropriate treatment. Please do not deal with this problem alone. Seek help from your health care provider, learn more about your problem, and use available resources as you take back control of this part of your life. If your motto has been "never pass up a rest room", keep reading this book and take action for yourself.

> *The shame is in*
> *not receiving*
> *appropriate treatment*

Bladder Works

Bladder works is not a hot topic in today's society. It is much more charming to talk about heart problems or knee repairs rather than bladder problems. No one hesitates to tell how many coronary arteries she has had bypassed or how many knee ligaments she has needed repaired after a skiing accident. This is usually followed by how she is progressing in her cardiac/knee rehabilitation program. It becomes a badge of courage and comparison with the next heart or knee patient. These people connect with a friendship and allegiance while in their "rehab" groups. They have "heart healthy" socials and become active in fund raising events. This camaraderie and support is great! But similar discussions about bladder control after delivery of the third baby or after a hysterectomy do not have the same visibil-

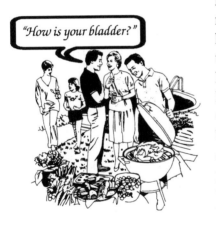

"*How is your bladder?*"

ity. Have you ever heard a new mother at a social even discuss how many pelvic muscle contractions she can now do and what is her current pelvic muscle strength level? (Or can you imagine an Olympic athlete discussing her bladder control problems after competition?) Do you know if your mother, aunt, sister or daughter has a bladder control problem? Probably not! It is not a subject frequently discussed.

Those of us involved in bladder works are not on the priority lists for social invitations because the host fears where the discussion will turn. ~DBS

When everything is working well, it is certainly appropriate to be discrete about urine, bladder, and elimination specifics. But when one has a problem, a discussion with a health professional is warranted. When approaching the problem, some degree of understanding will help.

Bladder

The bladder is a fascinating organ in its design and functional capabilities. It has the responsibility of storing and emptying urine on command from the brain. It is an organ composed of muscle fibers that can stretch as it fills with urine. It has three openings: two for ureters (tubes) that drain urine into the bladder from the kidneys; and one for the urethra (a tube that drains urine from the bladder to the outside of the body). At the base of the bladder there are valves or sphincters which remain closed to keep urine in the bladder and open to let the urine drain. When the bladder is full, the sphincters open and the bladder muscle contracts to force the urine out through the urethra.

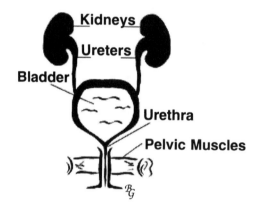

Urethra

The urethra is the tube that drains urine from the bladder to the outside of the body. It is a pliable, elastic, tubular organ that has several walls of thickness. The inner wall looks like folds with crevices. These crevices fill with secretions to make a better seal when the tube collapses for closure. The thickness, elasticity and moisture of the urethra are all important for a tight closure to keep urine from leaking.

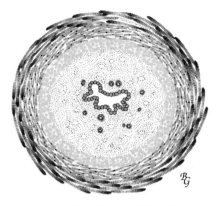

Cross Section of Urethra

In the female, the bladder lies just in front of the vagina, very close to the uterus. The urethra is short and exits in front of the vagina. The angle where the bladder joins the urethra is very important for urine control.

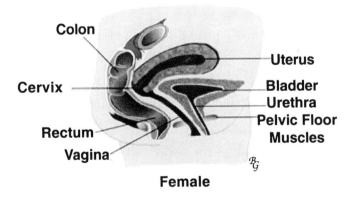

Female

Pelvic Muscles

Women have muscles and ligaments in the pelvic floor that provide support for the bladder and urethra, as well as the other pelvic organs. These muscles are affected by strengthening exercises, the amount of estrogen available, and forces that can stretch or stress them such as childbirth, surgery, and obesity.

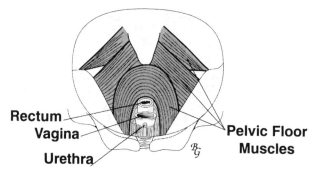

Rectum
Vagina
Urethra
Pelvic Floor
Muscles

Pelvic Floor Muscles

Nerve control

The nerve centers for emptying the bladder or inhibiting (delaying) the bladder from emptying are in the brain. The bladder sends a message to the brain signaling that the bladder is full of urine. The message to empty the bladder is then sent out from the brain, down through the spinal cord, branches off to peripheral nerves and goes to the bladder, sphincters, and surrounding pelvic muscles. These messages tell the sphincters or valves to relax and open and the bladder to contract and empty. It is a well-orchestrated event when everything is working correctly.

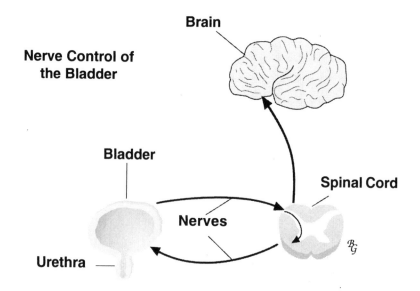

Nerve Control of the Bladder

Brain

Bladder

Spinal Cord

Nerves

Urethra

Bladder control is quite a complex event. Because so many parts of the body are involved, (the brain, spinal cord, branch nerves, blood vessels, bladder, urethra, hormones and pelvic muscles), there are numerous opportunities for some part or parts to work incorrectly.

This discussion may have seemed a little technical, but a brief overview is warranted so that the types and causes of incontinence can be explained. You can refer back to this section as needed.

Quiz - Did You Get It?

Match the following

1. ___ Urethra

2. ___ Incontinence

3. ___ Bladder

4. ___ Pelvic floor muscles

5. ___ Brain

a. support the bladder and urethra

b. stores urine

c. tube that drains urine to outside of body

d. loss of bladder control

e. control center for voiding

Correct answers: 1-c, 2-d, 3-b, 4-a, 5-e

ဢ *Chapter 2* ൙

Types of Incontinence

Types of Incontinence

Symptoms, risk factors and treatments vary according to the type of incontinence. This section includes information that will help you converse with your healthcare provider and better understand your role in dealing with these symptoms.

Transient Incontinence

There are some bladder control problems that are temporary, meaning that they are related to some other event or transient situation. These bladder control problems are not permanent. Other types of incontinence are chronic or long-term. The differences in these two types of incontinence are important to distinguish in order for treatment to be effective. The following are conditions or situations that can contribute to temporary or transient incontinence:

- bladder infection
- bladder stones
- some medications
- confusion or delirium
- restricted mobility
- depression
- dryness of the vagina and urethra (lack of estrogen)
- severe constipation

ᴥ large urine output (from diuretic medication, diabetes, congestive heart failure)

ᴥ spilling sugar (diabetes) or protein (kidney disease) in the urine

If the incontinence is related to any of the above conditions, correcting the causative problem may relieve the symptoms of incontinence. For example, treatment of a bladder infection can relieve incontinence related to bladder infection. When permissible, changing a medication that is contributing to incontinence may correct the incontinence. Once a confused patient with pneumonia and a high fever is no longer confused, incontinence events related to her confusion stop. Relieving severe constipation and reducing the pressure of the stool on the bladder and urethra can sometimes help urinary incontinence. Replacing the hormone estrogen in women can improve the dryness and elasticity of the urethra, increasing the urethra's ability to close tightly for better bladder control. It is so important to tell your health provider all of your symptoms so the appropriate treatment can be provided. For additional information, you may want to complete the assessment and severity index on pages 97-102 and give them to your healthcare provider as a record of your symptoms.

Personal Check List For You
Check the following conditions if you currently have them or have been treated in the past.

___ frequent bladder infections
___ bladder stones
___ arthritis, stroke or restricted mobility
___ depression
___ post-menopause (vaginal dryness)
___ routine constipation
___ prescribed diuretics
___ diabetes

Chronic Incontinence

Loss of bladder control or incontinence that is not related to a temporary situation is known as *chronic incontinence*. There are nu-

merous risk factors and causes of chronic incontinence. Being aware of them can often help to determine options that could minimize them. Factors contributing to chronic incontinence are covered below.

Aging

Although frequently considered to be related, incontinence is not a normal part of aging. It is not "a given" that everyone who ages will be incontinent. However, there are certain age-related changes or occurrences that can increase the risk of incontinence.

> *I am reminded of an elderly gentleman I met in a hospital lobby. He was limping and I asked him about his leg. He said his knee hurt. I asked if he had told his doctor. He said he had mentioned the pain to his doctor and that his doctor said it was due to old age. The gentleman wisely replied, "Doc, my other knee is just as old and it doesn't hurt". ~DBS*

There are factors that are associated with aging and can increase the risk of incontinence. They are as follows:

Decreased muscle tone-the bladder and pelvic floor muscles lose strength and tone. This would affect 1) the ability of the bladder to contract and empty and 2) the degree of support provided by the pelvic muscles to help the bladder sphincter close.

Increased bladder contractions, but with less strength-the bladder contracts more, but with less efficiency. It becomes more sensitive and hyperactive, but is not as effective as it contracts.

Decreased sensation-the nerves to the bladder are not as capable of carrying a message. The person is not as aware of the need to go to the bathroom or the message is delayed, so there is less time to move safely to the toilet without leaking urine.

Less mobility-the person requires more time getting to the bathroom and/or removing clothing after getting to the bathroom.

Decreased heart contraction strength-the heart is not as effective a pump as it once was. Because it cannot keep the blood moving through the body with the same force, fluids build up in the ankles and feet. This means there is less fluid available to circulate through the body and kidneys and less urine is made. This can lead to the next condition, increased urinary output at night.

Increased urinary output at night, or nocturia-there are fewer demands on the heart and circulation when one is lying at rest. Therefore, more blood flow is circulated to the kidneys and more urine is made. This results in a greater urinary output at night while the person is at rest, increasing the need for nighttime bathroom trips. (This one is related to decreased heart contraction strength as the cardiovascular system may not be able to pump enough blood to the kidneys during waking hours. When the latter occurs more blood goes to the kidneys during sleep, causing more urine to be made while at rest.)

Taking many medications at one time-some drugs may interact with one another or have side effects that affect bladder contractions (such as some sedatives or pain medicines) or sphincter release (such as some allergy, antihistamines or cold medications). The elderly are more likely to take multiple medications and be at a greater risk for interactions.

Co-existing ailments-a person may have diabetes and heart disease or Parkinson's at the same time. This usually means many symptoms and medications are interacting with one another.

Aging

A person's gender carries certain risk factors specific to that gender. As you will notice, women have many more risk factors for incontinence by virtue of their anatomy and childbearing abilities. And, corresponding to those risks, women have a greater incidence of urinary incontinence.

Female Risk Factors

The female pelvic floor has less structural strength than the male pelvic floor because the pelvic muscles are interrupted by the opening in the vagina. This affects the continuity and strength of the floor of muscles.

Pregnancy and childbirth put added stress on these muscles and on the bladder and its support structures. Women who have had multiple children or who have delivered large babies are more at risk for bladder control problems and pelvic floor relaxation because the tissues have had even greater stresses.

Hysterectomy, or surgical removal of the uterus, can increase the risk for incontinence. The uterus provides support to the bladder, to the urethra and to the important urethral-bladder angle. When the uterus is removed, these structures can "fall or lean" backwards to some degree. If they tilt out of position, the bladder and urethra may lose some of their ability to maintain continence.

Menopause results in a decrease in estrogen, the female hormone. Estrogen contributes to pelvic muscle and urethral strength. A decrease in estrogen can affect the strength of the supporting tissues for the bladder and the closing ability of the urethra.

Gender Risk Factors

Male	Female
prostate	pelvic floor structure
	pregnancy and childbirth
	hysterectomy
	menopause

Other Risk Factors

There are several disease conditions that can affect bladder control for both males and females.

Stroke-can interrupt the nerve messages from the brain to the bladder that are responsible for bladder control.

Diabetes-can cause an increase in the amount of urine produced, result in sugar spilling over in the urine, and can also affect the nerves and blood vessels involved in bladder functioning.

Parkinson's Disease-can affect messages from the brain needed for bladder control.

Alzheimer's Disease or other types of dementia-can affect the person's ability to remember how to use the toilet, where the toilet is located, or even what the toilet should be used for.

Multiple sclerosis-affects the spinal cord and can interrupt the nerve messages as they travel through the spinal cord.

Certain types of cancer and/or their treatments-various types of cancers, surgery or radiation treatments that involve organs in the pelvis, the brain, or spinal cord can influence bladder control by affecting the actual organ, its nerves or its blood supply. For example, treatment involving radiation to the pelvis for cancer of the cervix can affect the bladder and urethra because they are located so close to the cervix. Inflammation and later scarring to the tissues can occur with radiation treatments. Brain or spinal cord diseases or surgery can affect the nerve messages for bladder control. Cancer of the lung can result in chronic coughing and consequently, symptoms of stress incontinence.

Injury

Injuries can be very similar to diseases in their impact. Injuries to the spinal cord, brain, bladder or pelvis may result in disruption of

bladder control, depending on the areas affected. The actual organ itself may be injured or the nerves and blood vessels supplying the organ may be damaged, affecting the function of the organ.

Surgery

Surgeries of the bladder, urethra, brain, spinal cord, rectum, or other pelvic organs may interfere with some of the mechanisms for for bladder control in much the same way as an injury can, by causing trauma to the organ, supportive tissues, blood supply or nerve supply.

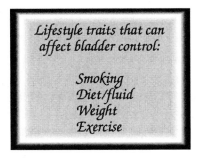

Lifestyle traits that can affect bladder control:

Smoking
Diet/fluid
Weight
Exercise

Lifestyle conditions

There are a few lifestyle traits that can increase the risk of incontinence. They include the following:

1. Smoking

Smoking can actually affect urinary incontinence in three ways. 1. Nicotine can be a bladder "irritant" causing the bladder to be more active, a situation that contributes to urge incontinence. 2. A smoker may have a chronic cough that increases abdominal pressure, weakens the bladder and urethral supports and contributes to stress incontinence. 3. Smoking can decrease the blood supply to the bladder by causing narrowing of the arteries.

2. Body mass or weight

Being overweight, or having a larger body mass, contributes to greater gravity forces on the pelvic muscles that support the bladder and urethra. This adds extra stress to the constant tone that the muscles must keep to support the pelvic organs. The muscles are more likely to stretch and offer less support.

3. Exercise

High-impact exercises (aerobics, jumping, jogging, physically active work or lifting) create more forceful stresses on the pelvic muscles and the support ligaments for the bladder. If the pelvic muscles have not been included in the exercise and strength training, the muscles of the abdomen get stronger and exert more force when they contract, while those of the pelvic floor are expected to take on this increased force without any site-specific training for them. The abdominal muscles contract with exertion, increase pressure on the bladder, yet the pelvic floor muscles have not been developed to counter this force.

4. Diet/fluid habits

Certain fluids and foods can be irritants to the lining of the bladder, causing the bladder to be sensitive and overactive. Some known bladder irritants are alcohol, caffeine, coffee, tea, soda, chocolate, spicy foods, citrus fruits and juices, tomatoes and tomato products, sugars, medicines with caffeine, milk, and artificial sweeteners (aspartame).

Note: Not everyone responds to each of these items the same. What may be a bladder irritant to one person might not be to another. The person has to observe which dietary products are causing urinary frequency and bladder irritability. By giving some attention to your response to food items, you can notice if a beer or a cup of coffee means a quick urine break for you. For some people, coffee may be an irritant and iced tea may not. It is an individual reaction.

By understanding how bladder control takes place as well as some of the causes or risk factors for incontinence, you may be able to either prevent incontinence, reduce your risk of incontinence, or reduce your incidents of incontinence. For example, if you

leak urine when you laugh or cough, you may be able to reduce those incidents by losing weight if you are heavy and/or by strengthening the muscles in your pelvic floor through pelvic muscle exercises. If you experience frequency of urination you may be able to reduce your frequency by eliminating bladder irritants from your diet and by altering your bladder habits.

Quiz: Did you get it?

Match the following

_____ 1. Pregnancy

_____ 2. Caffeine

_____ 3. Bladder infection

_____ 4. Hysterectomy

_____ 5. Lung cancer

_____ a. can be a bladder irritant

_____ b. surgical removal of the uterus

_____ c. can put added stress on pelvic floor muscles

_____ d. a common cause of transient incontinence

_____ e. can cause a chronic cough and urinary leakage

correct answers
1 - c, 2 - a, 3 - d, 4 - b, 5 - e

Types of Incontinence

Chronic incontinence is described as stress, urge, mixed, reflex, overflow, or functional. Brief descriptions, including risk factors, symptoms and treatment options, are discussed.

Stress Incontinence
Definition

Stress incontinence is a situation where urine leaks when there is some "stress" or force on the bladder from exertion or an increase in intra-abdominal pressure from events such as a sneeze or cough. Stress incontinence is related to a sphincter that does not close tightly, is not strong enough to tolerate increased pressures, or to inadequate support from the pelvic muscles.

Risk Factors

Women are more at risk because of the structure of their pelvic floor and with the vaginal opening through the pelvic floor muscles. Pregnancy, childbirth, obesity, high impact exercise, menopause, and chronic constipation increase the risk for stress incontinence.

Symptoms

Symptoms of stress incontinence may include leaking urine when lifting an object, laughing, coughing, sneezing, exercising, or even just rising from a sitting or lying position. Any of these activities can exert forces on the bladder which then transfer to the sphincter and allow urine to leak from the bladder.

Treatment Options
1. Behavioral Therapy

Behavioral therapy can be effective in a variety of ways for stress incontinence. Does the term *behavioral treatment* sound a little vague or unclear to you when you see it? Or have you had experience with behavioral treatments? You probably have and did not realize it. Behavioral treatment options are not new or vague. They are very precise and have been used quite effectively in many health situations.

> *Examples of behavioral treatments are diet changes, walking for exercise, emptying your bladder on a schedule or delaying an urge to go to the bathroom.*

Behavior is defined as how a person acts; the activities of a person, both physical and mental. Eating, walking, talking, writing, going to the bathroom, all of these are behaviors. Behavioral treatment options are those that affect a behavior or an activity that needs modification. Examples of behavioral treatments are diet changes, walking for exercise, emptying your bladder on a schedule or delaying an urge to go to the bathroom. Behavioral treatment options can be very specific and concrete. They involve an action or activity from the person. This is followed by learning appropriate behaviors AND persistence in incorporating the behaviors in one's life. **The person with the symptoms must make the effort!** The professional care provider can only provide education, guidance and support. Cardiac rehabilitation and knee therapy are both good examples of behavioral treatment options to restore strength and function. These are often used in conjunction with other therapies, such as surgery and medication, for an enhanced effect. The use of one does not preclude or eliminate the use of the other. Many times desired results are improved by combining the treatments. For example, with treatment of diabetes or heart disease, diet and exercise (both behavioral therapies) are often used in combination with medication for an enhanced effect.

What are the behaviors that you can use to help urinary incontinence?

You will be quite surprised at the number of behaviors that are safe and effective in helping with bladder control symptoms. Discuss them with your healthcare provider and incorporate those that

are appropriate for you in your lifestyle. You are never too young or too old to learn new behaviors, or to dismiss old behaviors. At my age, I am already thinking of health behaviors that I wish I had started at an earlier age.

> *Note: A few months ago my family adopted a lab puppy, a very social, loving, in-your-lap type creature. At four pounds, in-your-lap did not seem like such a big deal. Now, at 60 pounds, in-your-lap is not acceptable. But the puppy still likes it. When we started obedience training at 6 months, I learned that we had enforced a multitude of less-than-good behaviors that would now have to be corrected. I found myself wishing I had started correct training at 6 weeks, rather than 6 months. ~DBS*

2. Obesity

Eating habits can affect bladder symptoms through body weight. Obesity (excessive body mass) can increase the risk of both stress incontinence and urge incontinence. The extra weight of obesity increases the stress on the pelvic floor muscles. These muscles support pelvic organs (bladder, urethra and uterus) and abdominal organs against the pull of gravity the entire time the body is not lying down. Weight loss can reduce the forces against the pelvic muscles and lessen some of the stress. It can improve the symptoms of stress incontinence for some. Overweight women also have an increased risk for urge incontinence. The reason for this is not fully understood. It may be because of the increased abdominal pressure. Studies on urinary leakage and obesity have been done on women, but it may be possible that obese men are at greater risk for urinary leakage after prostate surgery than men of normal weight. Another reason to keep that body fit and trim! The scope of weight loss is beyond this book, other than for you to know it can be a factor in symptoms of stress incontinence in women. This book is about your pelvic floor and bladder health. Exercise and fitness specific to the pelvic floor muscles are very important to bladder control. Total body fitness and health should be considered in your goals.

3. Constipation

Constipation is quite common in the American lifestyle. You might wonder how is this relevant to urinary incontinence? Constipation, or hard formed stool in the rectum, can affect urinary function. If the rectum is filled with stool, pressure and forward displacement of the bladder can occur. This can affect the ability of the bladder sphincter to close tightly and prevent urine from leaking. A large amount of stool in the rectum can prevent the bladder from emptying completely. It can also aggravate an overactive bladder. Chronic straining (or bearing down) for bowel movement puts pressure on the pelvic floor muscles and can result in greater relaxation of the pelvic floor—similar to pushing down on a hammock and stretching it. Also, once the rectum fills with stool, an urge or message is sent out for bowel evacuation. If this urge is not responded to at that time, it is suppressed. If it is chronically suppressed, the urge

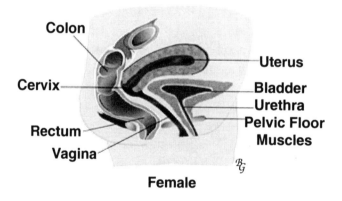

Female

becomes less noticeable and more easily ignored.

Several things can contribute to constipation, either temporarily or chronically. Medications, lack of exercise, a diet low in fiber and fluids, travel or change in routine, and illness can all contribute to constipation. If you have chronic problems with bowel elimination, you should consult your healthcare provider and begin a behavioral program for your bowels before you start a behavioral program for your bladder. This is important because your constipation can interfere with the effectiveness of your bladder program.

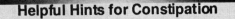

Helpful Hints for Constipation

1. Drink plenty of fluids
2. Eat grains, fruits and vegetables for fiber
3. Bran or fiber can be added to muffins, jam, cereal
4. Exercise daily
5. Try to establish a routine for bowel elimination
6. Respond to the urge for a bowel movement
7. Allow yourself plenty of time for evacuation
8. Avoid the use of laxatives if possible
9. See a healthcare provider experienced in bowel training programs

Jam recipe for constipation

The following is a recipe for a high fiber jam that can be made at home and kept in the refrigerator. Adding it to toast or crackers daily can help provide fiber to your diet and reduce constipation.

High Fiber Jam

1/2 cup Applesauce
1/2 cup Cooked dates/prunes/apricots
1/2 cup Bran

Flavor with 1 tbsp of your favorite jam. Mix together --it should be jam consistency. Keep refrigerated. Spread on toast or crackers daily. Adjust amount of jam or the amount of bran in the recipe depending on your need for relief of constipation. Drink plenty of fluids.

4. Pelvic Floor Muscle Strengthening

What and where are the pelvic floor muscles?

Pelvic floor muscles are the muscles in the pelvis that join with connective tissue (fasciae and ligaments) to support the bladder, rectum, urethra and uterus. The muscles are woven around the urethra like a web. Because the urethra has to close tightly to keep urine from leaking, the muscles around the urethra, when contracted, can help the urethra close tightly. These muscles also hold up (or support) your internal organs. Think of the floor of a house as a base foundation for the home. The pelvic floor muscles span the area between the sides of the pelvic bone. Just as electrical and plumbing lines run through a house floor framing, blood vessels and nerves run through the tissues of the pelvic floor. When you are standing, this floor of muscle support is similar to a hammock. A new hammock gives with weight, but still has stretch remaining and good support. An older and well-used hammock may tend to stretch and sag under weight. After pregnancy and childbirth, or with obesity, the pelvic floor muscles in women tend to relax and somewhat sag. After childbirth, few women actually learn to correctly exercise and rehabilitate this group of muscles, even though there may have been significant stretching and injury during the pregnancy, labor and delivery. Maintaining muscle tone and strength in these supportive tissues is very important for bladder control.

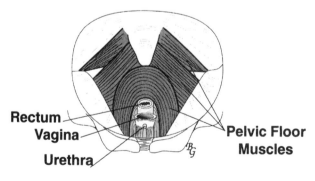

Rectum
Vagina
Urethra
Pelvic Floor Muscles

Pelvic Floor Muscles

There are two types of muscle fibers in the pelvic floor muscle group. Type I, or long muscle fibers, make up 70% of the muscle group and are responsible for sustained contractions. Type II, or short muscle fibers, make up the other 30% and are responsible for quick contractions such as those needed right before you sneeze. Think of the muscle fibers like runners—the long fibers are the distance runners (time and endurance); the short fibers are the sprint runners (fast and short acting). Both are needed for different circumstances of urinary control, therefore both should be strengthened.

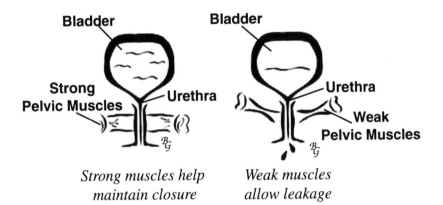

Strong muscles help
maintain closure

Weak muscles
allow leakage

How do you strengthen your pelvic floor muscles?

How does any muscle get stronger? Use, exercise and resistance. A muscle that is not used loses size, tone and strength. If you have ever had a cast on your leg or arm or were unable to use a limb because of injury or surgery, you probably noticed that the size of the muscle decreased from lack of use. The pelvic floor muscles keep some tone because they are in constant use supporting the pelvic and abdominal organs. But they do not develop optimum strength and endurance without active exercise and intentional contractions. Endurance is related to strength. Strength is the capacity of the muscle to contract, endurance is how long the muscle can maintain a capacity contraction. Both strength and endurance are needed to help with bladder support and control.

To develop strength in your pelvic muscles, you need to plan an exercise program. Just like any exercise program, goals needs to be set, a protocol followed, and effort consistently maintained. One problem is the difficulty in locating and correctly contracting the muscles in the pelvic floor. With a muscle in your arm, you can lift a two-pound weight and actually see the muscle contract. Note: it is difficult to do this with the pelvic floor muscles. You cannot see the muscles contract, so you have to learn the "feel" of the contraction. This is best done with biofeedback, either in-office or with a home unit. It is most important that you learn pelvic floor muscle exercises correctly before you start your protocol. Many women have thought they were doing correct muscle exercises (commonly called Kegels) only to conclude, "I did that, they did not help". Over 50 percent of women cannot perform a correct muscle exercise with verbal instructions alone. Doing pelvic muscle exercises incorrectly not only does not help bladder leakage symptoms, but can make the symptoms worse. It is worth your time and effort to get help in learning these exercises correctly.

The muscles in your pelvis go around your urethra, your vagina and your rectum. A correct contraction of these muscles is a motion of lifting up and in towards your body. It is as if you were going to stop your stream of urine or prevent gas from passing from your rectum. It is not a pushing-down movement. Many women have the tendency to also contract the muscles of the abdomen, thighs, or buttocks when trying to contract the pelvic muscles. Focus on keeping those muscles relaxed. You may want to lie down while you are learning, relax your body, take some deep breaths, and use biofeedback if possible. Become aware of the muscles that contract. Take deep breaths, exhale and contract. It is not easy to bear or push down with your abdominal muscles while you are exhaling. So you may want to practice breathing out while lifting the pelvic floor muscles.

Many women are told that they can practice these exercises anywhere, such as at a traffic light or while watching television. This may be true after some practice, but initially, learning the correct method requires concentration and focus. Consider your exercises in phases: the starter phase, the growth phase, and the maintenance phase.

Starter Phase

You may require several sessions to become aware of how a pelvic muscle contraction feels, and to eliminate the contractions of other muscles, such as those in

> *Consider this exercise a relaxation experience rather than a "work" effort.*

your abdomen or buttocks. Placing your hand on your abdomen while you are practicing will help you to be aware if those muscles are tense. Do not hold your breath; keep breathing while you exercise. Avoid having performance goals in your starter phase and focus on relaxing and learning the correct form. This is the phase where you focus on your pelvic floor muscles and get your body comfortable with the correct exercise. Learn to make relaxation a part of your exercise. Focus on your body parts, i.e. arms, legs, forehead, let them relax. Then focus on your pelvic muscles, where they are, what they feel like, how it feels to make them move. Breathing in and out slowly, listening to music, or mentally visualizing a tranquil setting can aid relaxation. Consider this exercise a relaxation experience rather than a "work" effort.

Pelvic Muscle Exercise Protocol

After you feel comfortable with your effort to contract the correct muscle, start your exercise protocol.

ᴥ Choose a comfortable place to exercise. Many women start by lying down, on their back with knees slightly bent (not fully) and feet flat on the surface. Some find that a small, flat pillow under the buttocks is comfortable. Some lie on their side. Others prefer to sit or stand. Eventually you will want to be able to correctly perform your contractions while in the car, at work, or even while doing an exercise activity such as swinging a golf club or just before a sneeze.

ᴥ Relax your body. Breathe deeply. Focus on your pelvic muscles.

ᴥ Pull your pelvic floor up and in toward your body. Do not strain

down. Hold this contraction for up to 10 seconds. Most will be able to hold a contraction for only one or two seconds in the beginning. Set your goal for holding the contraction for 5 seconds, then increase to 10 seconds as you get stronger.

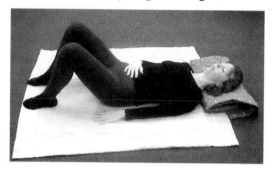

⋐ Do 10 contractions, taking a 10 second relaxation period between each contraction. Contract as hard as you can to begin developing strength. Holding the contraction for up to 10 seconds helps to develop endurance. When you start don't be discouraged if you can only hold a contraction for one or two seconds.

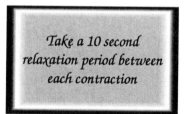

Take a 10 second relaxation period between each contraction

⋐ At the end of each session, do 10 quick contractions of your muscles. Contract and then totally relax the muscles within 1 to 1 1/2 seconds. These are important so you can develop the quick sprint muscles needed when you step out in the cold or just before you sneeze or laugh. Do not neglect this part of your exercise. These muscles (short, sprint fibers) are important.

⋐ Do two to three sessions a day. If your muscles get sore, you may need to cut back your sessions initially and work up more gradually.

❧ Do not overdo your exercises. The muscles may fatigue, become sore and your symptoms may get worse. (Just like your leg muscles may be sore after a long bike ride). Some women may feel discomfort in those muscles initially and some may have pain on intercourse for a short period of time. This will resolve after a few days of rest. Be sure to relax fully between your contractions. If you feel like you need a day off, take it. But be sure to continue your program. Skipping several days will result in loss of strength and endurance. When you return to your program, do not try to "catch up" by doing more exercises. Continue with your initial program.

It is not helpful to start off "gung ho" with 100 exercises a day, although some may believe that "more is better". This will not help relieve your bladder control symptoms any sooner. Plan a program and build muscle strength gradually as you would 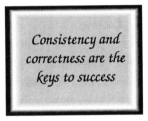 with any muscle strengthening program. Then stick with it.

As with any muscle exercise program, it takes time for your muscles to get stronger. It is doubtful that you could begin pelvic floor muscle exercises this week and be dry by next week. Don't we wish! Progress comes gradually. It will take several weeks of exercise before an improvement in symptoms will be noticed for most. Be patient. Consistency and correctness are the keys to success.

Growth Phase

This is the phase where you concentrate on progress. Improvements in muscle strength require resistance and overload. Resistance comes from contracting the muscles against an opposing force. Biofeedback with pneumatic sensors or vaginal cones can provide resistance. Overload refers to pushing the muscle to contract harder. While you are exercising, contract your muscle as hard as you can and hold the contraction for as long as you can, up to 10 seconds. You may start with very short contraction times, but with repetitions, you will

see progress. Your progress will come in increments and will not be a steady improvement. The day's events and your fatigue or energy levels will affect your performance at each session.

Maintenance Phase

After your symptoms have improved, you will need to continue doing these exercises in a maintenance format (i.e. once a day for 5 days/week) if you want to maintain the benefits from having strong muscles.

5. Biofeedback

Biofeedback was mentioned earlier. But what is it? It may sound very "vague" and not too scientific. To the contrary, biofeedback is widely used and accepted in clinical medicine. Biofeedback is simply an indicator or measure of a body's function or response that is not otherwise apparent. It is likely that you have one or more biofeedback devices in your home. Taking a person's temperature (thermometer) or blood pressure (blood pressure cuff) requires biofeedback. Standing on the scale for a measure of weight is biofeedback. People with diabetes use biofeedback (a glucometer) to test the sugar level of their blood.

Biofeedback is extremely useful in performing pelvic muscle exercises. Pelvic muscle exercises are not difficult to perform, but they can be difficult to learn correctly. If done incorrectly, pelvic muscle exercises can actually make your urinary symptoms worse. Having access to biofeedback can be a great coach for performing correct pelvic muscle exercises. It can be used to ensure a correct contraction, to maximize the contraction effort by showing the strength of the contraction, to show progress in strength and endurance of the muscle contraction, and provide motivation. All of this feedback is immediate during the exercise. A woman can see what her effort is producing before she is aware of symptoms improving. This provides encouragement and motivation to continue by giving feedback of her progress.

Biofeedback for urinary incontinence is available in office or clinic settings or home use. It is safe, effective, and does not cause any pain or discomfort. Generally, biofeedback is done by a clinician

using sensors to relay readings of your muscle contractions to the biofeedback equipment. The biofeedback tells you and the clinician if you are exercising correctly, how strong your contraction is, and how long the contraction lasts. It is very helpful in showing correct exercises and progress. This is usually done once a week for 4 to 6 office visits. A portable home biofeedback unit, *fria*®, is now available over-the-counter for pelvic muscle exercises. It is very economic and can provide the necessary biofeedback in the privacy of your own home. *fria* can be used with each exercise session, immediately feeding information back to the user about progress, strength and endurance. A home biofeedback unit is very much like an exercise trainer such as a treadmill, nordic track, or exercycle that gives feedback to you on your pulse rate, calories burned, distance, and/or speed. You become aware of where you are when you start the program, set goals, and see measurable progress along the way to achieving your goals.

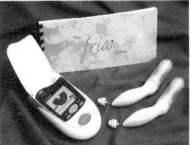

fria® **Home Biofeedback**
Courtesy of DesChutes Medical Products, Inc.
1011 SW Emkay Drive, Suite 104
Bend, OR 97702

How To

After consultation with your healthcare provider, lease or purchase a home biofeedback unit. Many of the manufacturers provide established exercise protocols for you. If not, use the following sample protocol.

❧ Commit to two five-minute sessions of pelvic muscle exercises a day.

❧ Select a time when you can relax and not be interrupted. For example, just after your bath or shower or while doing AM and PM hygiene.

❧ While you are learning, lie on the bed, floor, or sofa-get comfortable. Relax your body and focus on your pelvic floor muscles. Placing a small pillow under your lower back and slightly bending your knees may help. Some people prefer to lie on their side. Select a comfortable position.

❧ Set up your biofeedback unit and sensors.

❧ Take deep breaths for relaxing and concentrate on your exercises.

❧ Contract your pelvic floor muscles as hard as you can, holding the contraction for up to 10 seconds. Do not hold your breath. Keep breathing and contract your muscles on an exhale (breathe out).

> *If you do get away from your goals and off of your exercise schedule, review your goals and start again. Do not give up. This is for your own benefit. You are worth the few minutes a day that this takes to help decrease your bladder control symptoms.*

❧ Use your biofeedback unit to see the strength and length of your contraction.

❧ Periodically place your hand on your abdomen or your buttock to remind yourself not to contract that group of muscles.

❧ Relax 10 seconds between each contraction. This is very important.

❧At the end of every session with long contractions, do 10 to 15 quick muscle contractions.

❧ Use your biofeedback trainer for every session until you are sure you are performing your exercises correctly. Then use it at least once daily until you see symptoms improve.

❧ Record your biofeedback data daily by progress chart or diary. People who record their progress are twice as likely to continue their exercise.

> *People who record their progress are twice as likely to continue their exercises.*

❧ Set goals, today I want to reach a certain strength level or hold my contractions for a certain length of time. Combine these goals with fluid/food habits and urge suppression techniques. For example, today I will drink 7 glasses of water or today I will drink only one cup of coffee and I will try to suppress my urge to void for 15 minutes.

❧ Exercise at least 5 to 6 times a week. It is OK to skip a day every so often for rest. If possible, do not skip more than 3 or 4 days at a time or you will start to lose muscle strength and endurance.

Remember principles of muscle strengthening and exercise. Consistency and patience are required. Gains come in small increments. Your performance will not be the same every session. You may be tired during your afternoon session and not do as well. This is common. If you do get away from your goals and your exercise schedule, review your goals and start again. Do not give up. This is for

your own benefit. You are worth the few minutes a day that this takes to help decrease your bladder control symptoms. Make this just as routine as brushing your teeth.

6. Cones or Vaginal Weights

Vaginal cones or weights are available for female exercisers. They are cones that come in graduated weights and are shaped for vaginal insertion. Starting with the lightest weight cone, a woman inserts it in her vagina much like a tampon when she is going to perform her pelvic floor muscle exercises. This gives some resistance for the muscle to contract against. Over a few days, as her muscle gets stronger, she graduates to a cone with a greater weight, as someone would do who is lifting arm weights. After strengthening the muscle, she should try some exertion while the weights are in place, such as coughing or jumping. Just think of it as vaginal gymnastics! These cones weigh 20 to 70 grams. That does not sound like much, but you would not want to drop the heaviest one on your toe. A set of weighted vaginal cones can cost from $30 to $135. They should be made of a safe, smooth, medical grade material and cleaned thoroughly between each use. They are for one person to use and should not be shared with anyone else. You should not use them if you have a vaginal infection, irritation, or if they cause discomfort.

How To

Purchase a set of vaginal cones or weights. Follow the manufacturer's instructions for hygiene and insertion. A note of importance: exercising with the weights in place does little good if you are not performing the exercises correctly. It is very important to learn the proper technique. Work with your healthcare provider or with biofeedback to assure proper pelvic floor muscle exercise technique. Otherwise your exercise is ineffective and can even make your symptoms worse. This is like brushing your teeth when you have gum disease and recession of the gum tissues. If you continue with hard up-and-down brushing against the gums, the recession of the tissue gets worse. You have to learn the technique of brushing your teeth correctly in order to properly care for your gums.

If you are young, I encourage you to begin practicing healthy

bladder behaviors now, even if you do not have symptoms of urinary frequency or leakage. If you are already having symptoms of loss of bladder control, it is not too late to reverse some of the symptoms by starting behavioral treatment options. Most of these treatment options can be self-managed; some require professional assistance. Young or old, pass these ideas onto others that you care about.

7. Surgery

Surgery is very often used for stress incontinence in women. There are up to 200 variations of surgical procedures for female stress incontinence. You may have heard of some of them: anterior vaginal repair, bladder suspension, sling or specifically named for the physician credited to the procedure. Some very commonly used procedures are the Marshall/Marchetti/Krantz (MMK), Raz, Stamey, and the Burch procedure. Many of the surgical procedures are designed to add support for the position of the bladder and/or the urethra by tightening or anchoring the connecting tissues. These can add correction to the angle between the bladder and the urethra (important for continence in the female) and support for the bladder and urethra so they can work together for bladder control. Other procedures consist of injecting material (such as collagen) around the urethra to add bulk to help it close and seal more effectively. Another surgical procedure implants an artificial sphincter (cuff) or valve around the urethra that can be opened and closed as needed to let urine drain. Surgery may be necessary for you. Discuss this with your physician or practitioner. Be aware of your options and what you can do to work with your doctor to improve your results, no matter which therapy is used. If you do require surgery - prepare yourself for complete recovery. Do not lift, push, or strain with a bowel movement until totally healed. Start pelvic muscle exercises to add support. Behavioral options can always be combined with surgery and medications. Research has shown that pelvic muscle exercises increase effectiveness of surgery and medications.

8. Medications

There is no specific "pill" to take that will cure stress incontinence without experiencing some other effects. Medications are more

commonly used with urge incontinence than with stress incontinence because of the mechanism of the problem. But there are medications available that can help control symptoms in some people with stress incontinence. For those persons, this could make a major medical problem more acceptable. It varies with each person, as will all treatment options. Some medications affect the tone of the bladder neck and the urethra, some improve the strength of the sphincter closure. Basically they increase the resistance of the sphincter. Certainly discuss your options with your physician or practitioner.

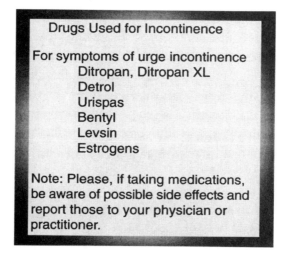

Drugs Used for Incontinence

For symptoms of urge incontinence
    Ditropan, Ditropan XL
    Detrol
    Urispas
    Bentyl
    Levsin
    Estrogens

Note: Please, if taking medications, be aware of possible side effects and report those to your physician or practitioner.

Urge Incontinence

Definition

This refers to a strong need (or urge) to go to the bathroom in a hurry. This can be quite uncomfortable and even painful. It is sometimes referred to as bladder instability, overactive bladder, or hypersensitive bladder. Your bladder is telling you that you need to empty it even though it is not full. With urge incontinence a very small amount of urine in the bladder can send a signal for the need to empty. Urge incontinence is the involuntary loss of urine associated with a strong urge or desire to go to the bathroom and inability to wait. The person receives a strong message to go to the bathroom, but has a very short time before the bladder contracts. Many times she cannot

delay the urge and avoid leaking urine. This may come in association with environmental situations such as stepping out in the cold; being near the freezer section of the grocery store; hearing, seeing or touching water; arriving home and knowing a toilet is near; or conversely, being on a trip and knowing a toilet is not near. Frequent urination at night is also associated with urge incontinence. Some have symptoms of urgency or frequency, going to the bathroom 20-30 times/day but leakage is minimal.

Normally, the bladder stores urine until it receives a message that it is full. The bladder then contracts, the sphincters responsible for closure open, and urine is eliminated. If not in a socially acceptable place for going to the bathroom, this message can be ignored and going to the bathroom delayed for awhile. These messages are relayed from the bladder, through the spinal cord, to the brain and back to the bladder and sphincters. Anything that disrupts the nerve paths carrying these messages can interfere with the bladder function and cause symptoms of urgency or bladder overactivity. In the simplest of terms, it means the person senses the need to go to the toilet, but cannot get there in time to avoid a leak.

Risk Factors

Urge incontinence can be related to a neurological event such as stroke or Parkinson's disease, but it can also exist because of bladder obstruction, stones, urinary tract infection, or an irritated bladder (the lining of the bladder is inflamed or irritated due to dietary intake or bacteria in the urine).

Symptoms

Symptoms include the following:

⮞ Having to go to the bathroom frequently

⮞ Feeling the need to go in a hurry (urgency)

⮞ Getting up at night several times to void

⮞ Responding to a repeated activity such as having to go to the

bathroom as soon as you put your key in the door to your home (a mental stimulus not necessarily related to a full bladder)

❧ Urge to go to the bathroom when stepping out in the cold or rain, hearing water running, or getting near the refrigerated section in the grocery store, even if your bladder was just emptied a few minutes earlier

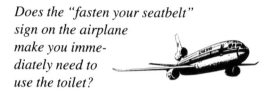

Does the "fasten your seatbelt" sign on the airplane make you immediately need to use the toilet?

It is not uncommon for a person with urge symptoms to be in the bathroom every 45 to 60 minutes. It can be extremely disruptive to anyone's lifestyle to always need to know where the next restroom can be found.

Treatment Options
1. Behavioral Therapy

Foods and fluids (type and amount) can affect your bladder symptoms. With information about how fluids and foods affect your symptoms you can choose diet and fluid intake behaviors which will allow you to better control your bladder symptoms. In Chapter 3, there is a 24/hour bladder and fluid habit sheet. Complete this form to learn what you are drinking, when and how much, how quick you must get to the toilet after a drink, and when you have bladder leakage in relation to what you drink. This is valuable information that will help you make decisions about behaviors to consider for improvement.

Do you view coffee as a "bladder enemy?"

Fluids

Why is fluid management of importance? Fluids are crucial to all functions of the body. They have a very big impact on how the bladder works, since a great deal of fluid elimination is via the bladder.

Many persons with loss of bladder control think that if they limit their fluid intake, they will have to go to the bathroom less and have less urine leakage. It is true that they will make less urine if they drink less, but this may actually increase their symptoms of bladder control. If a person has had too little to drink, the body conserves fluids by decreasing what the kidney and bladder will eliminate. As a result, the amount of urine decreases. As the amount of urine goes down, the urine becomes stronger or more concentrated.

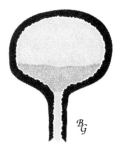

> *Think of making a pitcher of lemonade from a powder packet. If you only add half of the recommended water to the pitcher, the lemonade will be stronger and more concentrated than if you added the recommended amount. By adding more water you can dilute the lemonade.*

Just as concentrated lemonade may make your mouth "pucker", strong or concentrated urine can make your bladder "pucker" or contract. The bladder can react with strong contractions even though it is not full of urine. The concentrated urine enters the bladder, serves as a "stimulant" and gives the person a quick urge or need to get to the bathroom. The bladder contracts more actively than normal. Therefore, if you have tried to cut back on drinking fluids in an attempt to prevent leaking urine, you may actually have more urgency and leakage. Fluids are needed to keep the urine from becoming too concentrated. Women with symptoms of urge incontinence (frequency, having to get to the bathroom in a hurry) or mixed incontinence need to drink water throughout the day rather than in large amounts at a single time. Fluid restriction may be appropriate at the

end of the day a few hours before bedtime. But all-day fluid restriction, unless advised by your health professional for some other health condition, is not a healthy idea.

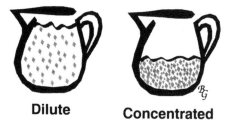

Dilute   Concentrated

The preferred way to drink fluids is to drink small amounts of liquid throughout the day. Cutting back on fluids leads to greater urine concentration. Drinking large amounts of fluid at one time causes a large amount to enter the bladder rapidly causing urgency and bladder contractions. The bladder functions better with fluid entering it gradually throughout the day. Today's "trend" of carrying a water bottle everywhere and sipping small amounts throughout the day is actually a very good behavioral option for bladder control problems.

Water is the most preferred type of fluid. Some fluids are "irritants" or "stimulants" when they reach the bladder. The mechanism of this action is not fully understood, but it is believed that "irritants" cause increased bladder activity, urgency and contractions. When the bladder lining is irritated, the person has to void more frequently, and usually in a hurry. Suspected bladder "irritants" are shown.

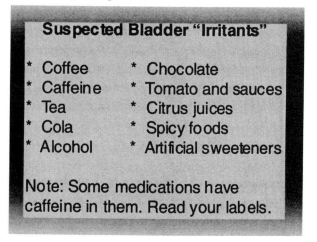

Suspected Bladder "Irritants"

* Coffee   * Chocolate
* Caffeine   * Tomato and sauces
* Tea   * Citrus juices
* Cola   * Spicy foods
* Alcohol   * Artificial sweeteners

Note: Some medications have caffeine in them. Read your labels.

Not everyone is affected the same by these "irritants". What bothers one woman may not affect another. It is an individualized response. You must observe your own reaction to various foods and drinks. One person reported an increase in urgency and frequency after ingesting Altoids, a common breath mint. If you suspect an item bothers your bladder, eliminate that item for a few days to see if you can observe a difference in your bladder habits. If your bladder is sensitive, it may take a few days without the item before a difference is noted. If you do find that coffee or chocolate or lemonade is an "irritant" it does not mean that you have to totally give up the item. But you may want to be selective in the timing of when you choose to take the item. For example, you may want to eliminate that item while on a plane ride or car trip, in the late afternoon, before church or a social function, or before a long business meeting.

Some fluids act as diuretics, meaning they increase urine output. After drinking a diuretic a person will soon have to empty the bladder. Known diuretics are water, beer, coffee, soda, watermelon, grapefruit juice, and tea. Again, pay attention to your personal reactions to what you are drinking and make your choices from that information. Be careful not to reduce your intake to a level that causes your body to conserve fluid and concentrate your urine. Six to eight glasses of water per day are generally recommended. If you are exercising, live in a dry, hot climate, or have a fever or diarrhea increase your water intake.

> *In a study of 450 female soldiers conducted by physicians in the Department of Obstetrics and Gynecology at Madigan Army Medical Center, Tacoma, WA, one third of the women experienced urinary incontinence during their exercise and field training activities. A disturbing fact was that thirteen percent of these women limited their fluid intake significantly to reduce their urinary symptoms.*[4]

Limiting fluids, or self-dehydrating, during exercise can be very dangerous. It should not be done. Dehydration cannot only result in

low urine output but can cause dizziness, confusion, irritability, heat exhaustion, and even coma. Extreme dehydration can lead to death. If you are exercising, keep up your fluid intake. One rule of thumb is to drink enough fluids that your urine is very lightly colored or almost clear.

Your fluid habits
Check the following that you drink and estimate an amount. *Review your 24-hour fluid sheet.*

Drink/ingredient	Cups per day
_____water	_____
_____caffeinated coffee	_____
_____decaffeinated coffee	_____
_____cola	_____
_____tea	_____
_____alcohol	_____
_____cocoa	_____
_____citrus juice	_____
_____tomato juice	_____
_____lemonade	_____
	Packets/day
_____artificial sweeteners	_____

Diet
How does diet affect bladder habits?

Food derivatives that are eliminated in the urine can affect the bladder. When the derivative of an "irritant" is eliminated through the bladder, the bladder will actively contract with urgency before it has completely filled with urine. This creates the urge to urinate, often in a hurry. Foods that can have this affect on some people are

chocolate, spicy foods, citrus fruits, and tomatoes. Fluids and foods that may be irritants, is a very individual matter. What may be an irritant to one person's bladder may not affect another. It takes observation of the food intake and the bladder's response to determine which foods, if any, may cause bladder urgency.

Your Food Habits

Check the following foods if you eat them frequently (more than three times a week). If you suspect a problem with any of the fluids or foods, you may want to keep a 7-day fluid/food diary and note your response of bladder symptoms. Do they improve with elimination of certain foods? Do your symptoms return when you re-introduce a certain food or fluid? Start by eliminating the food or fluid you suspect for 7 to 10 days. Give it enough time for your bladder irritation to resolve. Then reintroduce the item and see if your bladder urgency or frequency recurs or gets worse.

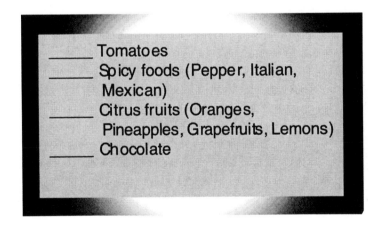

_____ Tomatoes
_____ Spicy foods (Pepper, Italian, Mexican)
_____ Citrus fruits (Oranges, Pineapples, Grapefruits, Lemons)
_____ Chocolate

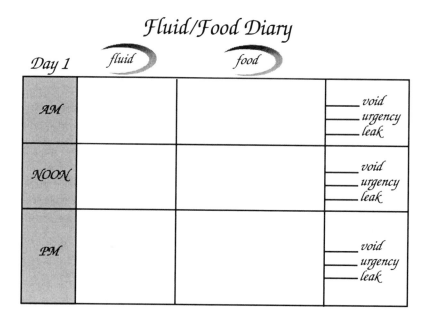

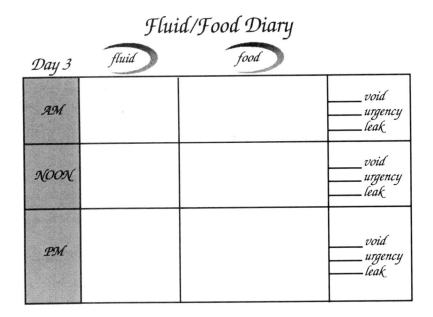

Fluid/Food Diary

Day 3   *fluid*   *food*

	fluid	food	
AM			_____ void _____ urgency _____ leak
NOON			_____ void _____ urgency _____ leak
PM			_____ void _____ urgency _____ leak

Fluid/Food Diary

Day 4   *fluid*   *food*

	fluid	food	
AM			_____ void _____ urgency _____ leak
NOON			_____ void _____ urgency _____ leak
PM			_____ void _____ urgency _____ leak

Fluid/Food Diary

Day 5 *fluid* *food*

	fluid	food	
AM			_____ void _____ urgency _____ leak
NOON			_____ void _____ urgency _____ leak
PM			_____ void _____ urgency _____ leak

Fluid/Food Diary

Day 6 *fluid* *food*

	fluid	food	
AM			_____ void _____ urgency _____ leak
NOON			_____ void _____ urgency _____ leak
PM			_____ void _____ urgency _____ leak

Fluid/Food Diary

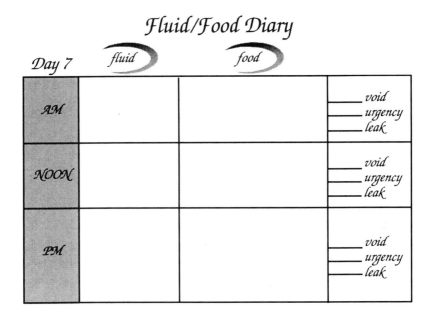

Day 7	*fluid*	*food*	
AM			_____ void _____ urgency _____ leak
NOON			_____ void _____ urgency _____ leak
PM			_____ void _____ urgency _____ leak

Pelvic Muscle Exercises/Biofeedback

Pelvic muscle exercises and biofeedback are very effective with urge incontinence. These take time to make improvements; patience and motivation are required. Side effects are all but non-existent. Pelvic floor muscle re-education can be used to inhibit the sacral nerve reflex that causes the bladder to contract. By correctly squeezing the pelvic floor muscles, the bladder is given a message to relax.

See how to perform theses exercises under treatment options for stress incontinence. Bladder training and urge suppression techniques can be helpful for urge incontinence.

Bladder Training

Bladder training may sound sort of athletic or military. It is also referred to as bladder drill, which gives even more of a military picture. It does require some regimen to be effective. But don't knock this concept. It can be helpful.

Some women have been taught to empty their bladder frequently to prevent urinary stasis. This has been particularly true for women with frequent urinary tract infections. Eventually the bladder becomes "trained" to not store as much urine as before. The bladder develops a smaller capacity to hold urine and requires more frequent voids, every 30 minutes, every 45 minutes, etc. This can be disruptive, especially if the frequency occurs through the night.

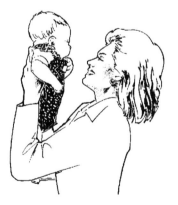

Sally is a 33-year-old mother of two. She has to urinate frequently in the daytime, every 45 minutes and sometimes as frequent as every 15 minutes. Sometimes she feels like she needs to urinate again as soon as she finishes. She is a professional in the healthcare field and finds this frequency to be very disruptive at work. She does not leak urine, but starts to feel very uncomfortable if she does not empty her bladder frequently. She drinks several cups of coffee every morning and 2 to 3 sodas (diet/caffeine free) throughout the day. Sally sought help for

her urinary frequency and was recommended for behavioral therapy.

Sally's first behavior modification was her fluid intake. She gradually began to reduce her coffee and soda intake and increase her water intake. Her goal was to reduce the fluid irritants to her bladder allowing it time to settle down and become less hyperactive.

Her next behavior was to practice letting her urge pass by using urge suppression and waiting 15 minutes before going to void. She was careful not to wait too long. Her goal was to gradually increase her bladder's capacity.

Sally was, in effect, working on bladder training and fluid modification. She started to see improvements within four weeks and was able to wait 2 hours between voids by 8 weeks. Her goal was to reach 2.5 hours. This may not seem like much, but to one who was constantly thinking about the bathroom, this was a major accomplishment for her.

Bladder training may appear quite simple, so much that you may minimize its capabilities to help your symptoms improve. Remember, the bladder is a muscle and it works in response to a message sent by a nerve. To start any type of muscle/nerve training you have to deliberately think, then act, and practice repeatedly. Eventually, the "think" part becomes almost subconscious and it is more like a "reaction". Think of learning to use a typewriter or a computer keyboard (if you did). Initially every letter required the thought of "what is the letter?", "where is it located?", "which finger should I use?". After time and practice, the mind and fingers react almost as one with the fingers finding the correct letter in rapid time. Perhaps if you didn't learn to type, you may have learned to dribble a basketball. Again, in the beginning you have to look at the ball, think about your hand and the dribble. After time and practice it becomes a reaction, the ball goes with you, bouncing up and down on the floor as you run. Can a bladder be "trained"? In a manner of speaking, yes. The bladder can be "trained" to suppress an urge to empty, to hold more urine, or to empty more completely.

Decide what symptoms you want to improve, what you want your bladder "trained" to do. Do you want to go to the bathroom less frequently? Are you emptying your bladder every 45 minutes? Are you

getting up in the night 4 or 5 times to go to the bathroom? Do you have to go to the bathroom 15 minutes after you just went because you do not completely empty your bladder? Write out some of the symptoms that you have and goals related to each symptom. Record your progress by week as you work on each symptom. Here are some training protocols.

SYMPTOMS I HAVE

Example 1: *I have to go to the bathroom every hour while awake.*
Example 2: *As soon as I walk in my house, I have to rush to the bathroom.*

1._____
2._____
3._____
4._____
5._____

GOALS

Example 1: *I want to delay going to the bathroom 15 minutes.*
Example 2: *I want to slowly enter my home and wait 10 minutes before going to the toilet.*

1._____
2._____
3._____
4._____
5._____

MY PROGRESS

Week 1

1._____
2._____
3._____
4._____
5._____
6._____

Week 2

1._____
2._____
3._____
4._____
5._____
6._____

Week 3

1._____
2._____
3._____
4._____
5._____
6._____

Week 4

1._____
2._____
3._____
4._____
5._____
6._____

Week 5

1._____

2._____

3._____

4._____

5._____

6._____

Week 6

1._____

2._____

3._____

4._____

5._____

6._____

Week 7

1._____

2._____

3._____

4._____

5._____

6._____

Week 8

1._____

2._____

3._____

4._____

5._____

6._____

How To

Train the bladder to not have to empty so frequently.

Problem: I need to go to the bathroom almost every hour, even more frequently in the morning after my coffee.

Fact: I urinate an average of 17 times a day. I drink two cups of regular coffee every morning and one cup in the late afternoon. (noted on my bladder/fluid habit sheet)

Goal: I would like to reduce the number of times I have to urinate to 12 a day.

Approach:

Urge Inhibition or Suppression

You will need to know how to correctly perform a pelvic muscle contraction. This is where your quick pelvic muscle contractions will help. This process requires practice and time to succeed. Do not make the mistake of thinking that if you do this one time correctly, you will be safe. Practice it in a comfortable environment with a toilet nearby until you have control.

When you get an urge to urinate, take a deep breath, relax, then perform a quick pelvic muscle contraction and let the urge pass. Distract yourself mentally if you can. Try a brief physical distraction such as putting up the dishes, making out a to-do list, straightening up your desk, or making a quick phone call. During your distraction, keep relaxing by taking slow, deep breaths. This becomes easier the more you practice.

The urge usually will pass in just a few seconds. You have been doing this all of your life when you have needed to pass gas or have a bowel movement, yet the setting was not appropriate. You "suppressed the urge" until you were in a suitable place. Children, often waiting until the last minute to give the warning that they need to go to the bathroom, have to learn to suppress an urge while mom frantically looks for a toilet. ~DBS

Wait a few minutes, then slowly move to the toilet. Rushing only makes the bladder more likely to contract more. This increases the chance of an "accident", either leaking urine or falling down.

Each time you need to void, try to increase the minutes that you delay going to the toilet. Increase the time by whatever you feel comfortable with in terms of getting to the toilet without leaking. At first it may be 5 minute intervals, then 15 minutes. Gradually increase to having a 2.5 to 3 hour interval. It may take up to a week to increase your time to even 15 minutes. If you have severe urge symptoms, it may take even longer. Try to not get discouraged. Be patient and keep practicing.

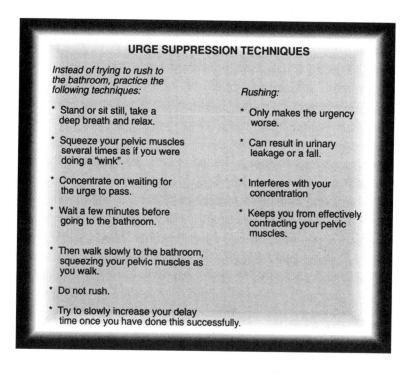

URGE SUPPRESSION TECHNIQUES

Instead of trying to rush to the bathroom, practice the following techniques:

Rushing:

* Stand or sit still, take a deep breath and relax.

* Squeeze your pelvic muscles several times as if you were doing a "wink".

* Concentrate on waiting for the urge to pass.

* Wait a few minutes before going to the bathroom.

* Then walk slowly to the bathroom, squeezing your pelvic muscles as you walk.

* Do not rush.

* Try to slowly increase your delay time once you have done this successfully.

* Only makes the urgency worse.

* Can result in urinary leakage or a fall.

* Interferes with your concentration

* Keeps you from effectively contracting your pelvic muscles.

Avoid Bladder Irritants

Because bladder irritants may be making your bladder more sensitive and active while you are trying to calm the bladder muscle, discovering and eliminating those drinks or foods that are irritants can be a big help in bladder training. Decreasing your coffee or

caffeine intake may or may not help, but it is worth investigating to see if it makes a difference.

2. Surgery

Surgery is used more often for stress incontinence than for urge incontinence. That is because stress incontinence is frequently related to structural problems and urge incontinence is more related to the nerve impulses to the bladder or to something irritating the lining of the bladder. However, there is a surgical procedure for severe cases of urge incontinence where a device is implanted that provides electrical stimulation to inhibit the sacral nerve and reduce impulses to the bladder. This is known as neuromodulation. Neuromodulation is new and is being used by urologists to treat urge incontinence that has not responded to conventional treatments. It is a surgical procedure used in a select population of people with overactive bladder or chronic pelvic pain that have not responded to other less invasive treatment. This form of treatment is in its early stages of clinical use and is considered a promising treatment for selected patients.

3. Medications

Medications are frequently used to treat urge incontinence. Medications designed to inhibit the nerve paths to the bladder can be effective in reducing the activity (or overactivity) of the bladder. Many persons have been helped by this mode of therapy. Some of the medications do have side effects such as dry mouth, dry eyes, drowsiness or constipation and are contraindicated in patients with uncontrolled glaucoma. These may reduce patient comfort and compliance. Sometimes medications are used to decrease symptoms while the patient begins a course of behavioral therapy. Not everyone is a candidate for these medications. Again, discuss this option with your physician or nurse practitioner.

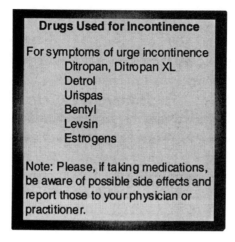

Drugs Used for Incontinence

For symptoms of urge incontinence
  Ditropan, Ditropan XL
  Detrol
  Urispas
  Bentyl
  Levsin
  Estrogens

Note: Please, if taking medications, be aware of possible side effects and report those to your physician or practitioner.

4. Electrical Stimulation

Electrical stimulation or E-stim, as it is frequently called, sounds quite scary. Who wants to have their bladder stimulated! Actually, it is a barely perceptible stimulation of the pelvic floor muscles to cause a contraction of the muscles. It is sometimes used in conjunction with pelvic floor muscle exercises. The clinician uses the E-stim to help the patient learn the location of the pelvic floor muscles and to get accustomed to the sensation of a contraction. This helps the patient learn to contract the muscles correctly. This procedure is done in an office or clinic setting. Some clinicians use E-stim to help the person correctly learn pelvic floor muscle exercises, some use it as a passive method of muscle contraction. E-stim may be slightly uncomfortable, but not painful. It is most effective when done in conjunction with correct pelvic muscle exercises on a consistent basis. E-stim treatment is performed in a clinical setting with a trained healthcare provider.

5. Spinal Neuromodulation (or sacral nerve stimulation)

A form of electrical stimulation can also be delivered by implanting a small device that applies short bursts of electrical currents to certain nerves that affect bladder contractions. This is a surgical procedure and is used in a select population of people with overactive bladders or chronic pelvic pain that have not responded to other less invasive treatments.

6. Electromagnetic Therapy

Electromagnetic innervation is a term used for a new technology using pulsed magnetic fields to stimulate the nerves and muscles and cause the pelvic floor muscles to contract. There is no electric current or pain that makes the patient feel uncomfortable. It is a passive method of causing the muscles to contract. This therapy is done in a clinic or office setting and requires multiple appointments.

Mixed Incontinence

Definition

Mixed incontinence is a combination of stress and urge incontinence. It is very common in women and becomes more common as one ages.

Risk Factors

Risk factors are those included with stress and urge incontinence. At particular risk are older females who have had children, are on multiple medications, and have had a stroke, diabetes, or Parkinson's Disease.

Symptoms

Women may have an urgent or frequent need to go to the bathroom as well as leaking urine with a laugh, sneeze, cough, lift, or exercise.

Treatment Options
1. Behavioral Therapy

Behavioral therapy is a very good option for mixed incontinence because it addresses the causative mechanics of both stress and urge incontinence. Diet and fluid therapy, urge suppression techniques, bladder training, pelvic floor muscle exercises, and biofeedback all work to reduce symptoms of mixed incontinence. They are presented under stress and urge incontinence.

2. Surgery

Surgery, at present, is more specific for stress incontinence. A surgical procedure that may relieve stress incontinence symptoms would only relieve the mixed incontinence symptoms if they are related to the stress incontinence. Surgery to implant a neurostimulating device would only improve the urge symptoms.

3. Medications

Medications are generally more useful for urge incontinence. A person with mixed incontinence may benefit from the combination of surgery and medications.

Reflex Incontinence

This is usually related to a spinal cord or nerve injury. The timing of the bladder contraction and the sphincter opening are uncoordinated. The bladder and the sphincter may contract at the same time, resulting in painful obstruction of the flow of urine. The person may not even feel the need to void, yet the bladder can overfill and then leak.

1. Surgery

Surgery may be used to relieve the closing function of the sphincter. This would allow urine to flow continuously and some type of containment management would be needed. There are also surgical procedures to reconstruct bladder-type organs or divert the urine into an external pouch.

2. Medications

Medications may be used to relax the bladder and prevent spasms or to relax the sphincters.

Overflow Incontinence

Definition

The bladder becomes too full and then leaks small amounts of urine as the bladder pressures rise.

Risk Factors

In women it may be associated with a urethral stricture (narrowing). It also may occur after surgery for bladder suspension. It can also be associated with diabetes.

Symptoms

Symptoms include difficulty starting a urine stream, having to strain to use the bathroom, voiding a small amount and having to go back to the bathroom again in a few minutes.

Treatment Options

1. Behavioral Therapy

Double voiding is helpful in some cases of overflow incontinence. Double void, this is a term your healthcare person may say to you and you think "what does that mean?" It means just what it says, empty your bladder twice.

How To

Go to the bathroom the first time, relax your bladder just a few seconds, then try to empty your bladder again. For the second attempt, it may be helpful to change position, lean forward, or press above your bladder with your hand. Some walk around the room or move around just a little Many times, the second attempt produces more urine than the first. This is very common as one gets older. Double voiding can be very helpful for persons who are not emptying their bladder completely the first time. It takes very little time and is certainly worth adding to your toileting habits to see if it helps.

> *Interestingly enough, this is something many pregnant women learned to do without even thinking about it, changing positions on the toilet and straining a second time to eliminate more urine. Being pregnant with a baby sitting on the top of the bladder has a way of distorting the shape of the bladder and the urethra. ~DBS*

2. Medications

Medications are now available that can reduce the resistance of the sphincter. Discuss these options with your healthcare provider.

3. Surgery

Surgery may be used to relieve the obstruction. Depending upon the cause of the obstruction surgery may remove the obstruction or dilate the urethral opening. Laser, microwave and cryo (freezing) surgery techniques are available as well as traditional "cutting" methods to remove an obstruction.

Functional Incontinence

Definition

This does not refer to any problem with the urinary system as such. It occurs when there are functional barriers that make it difficult to reach a toilet. By taking away access to a toilet, anyone, under certain circumstances, can become functionally incontinent. This is a very common type of incontinence in the elderly, but anyone can experience functional incontinence. See the excerpt below and see if you can identify.

Note: The following is taken from Dr. Pat D. O'Donnell's medical textbook titled Urinary Incontinence. The quote is from Chapter One called The Personal Side of Incontinence, written by Dr. Tamara Bavendam, a urologist, and Cheryle Gartley, founder of the Simon Foundation for Continence, US.

> *"It took 3 cups of coffee to hang in there, but the meeting is finally over. My next appointment is across town in 30 minutes-manageable if there are no delays. I need to "go", but time is tight-no big deal—I'll go when I get there.*
>
> *Traffic is unbearably slow and then comes to an abrupt standstill just before the bridge. I'll be late for my appointment—thank goodness for my cellular phone. If I had only known there was going to be a delay, I*

would have stayed and used the bathroom.
The urge is increasing. Is there any way of getting out
of traffic and finding a bathroom? No!

Thinking of other things helps. Concentrate on the
radio—it's not so bad...Fifteen minutes later the traf-
fic is thankfully moving. Where is the nearest bath-
room? Just thinking about a bathroom makes the urge
become overwhelming, almost painful. 'What if I don't
get to the bathroom soon? Will my bladder rupture?
Will I wet my pants? Don't think about it; just drive!'
A gas station ahead on the right. Great! Just cross
the three lanes of traffic and I'm home free. The urge
and spasms are building every second. There's a con-
stant throbbing sensation I can't ignore.

Screech! Slam on the breaks! Where did that idiot
come from? At least I didn't get hit! Wait, why am I
feeling warm? I WET MYSELF-#X@!X%z@!! Now
what am I going to do?"

This is followed by this comment from the authors of the chapter:

"The scenario described above is not a personal fail-
ure, nor does it mean anything is malfunctioning with
the lower urinary tract. The involuntary loss of urine
was the expected outcome that particular set of cir-
cumstances where the limits of the bladder and the
bladder-outlet mechanism were reached and ex-
ceeded. The sudden distraction of the 'near accident'
and 'slamming' on the brakes allowed the develop-
ing bladder contraction to overcome the forces of the
sphincter mechanism."[5]

> *The more regularly you exercise your pelvic floor muscles, the greater the benefits of bladder control and pelvic support*

Risk Factors

Typical barriers, other than the situational one described above, that may prevent or delay access to a toilet are as follows:

ى Problems with mobility such as an injury (broken ankle), surgery (knee or hip surgery), or illness (flu, pneumonia)

ى Difficulty with dexterity or hand movements that could interfere with removing clothing for toileting (arthritis, Parkinson's, or weakness from a stroke)

ى Problems with mental capability such as Alzheimer's or other types of memory impairment (cannot find/recognize the toilet).

Barriers can also be environmental, such as the distance to the toilet or shared use of a toilet; poor lighting available for the toilet; tight clothing that is difficult to remove; an intravenous (IV) tub- 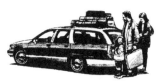 ing and pole; side rails pulled up on the bed while in the hospital; or simply being in an unfamiliar environment at night, waking with a need to void, but not fully able to negotiate an unfamiliar route without an accident. It is not uncommon for a youngster or an elderly woman to visit a relative and have a nighttime accident (loss of bladder control) because the environment in unfamiliar. This is terribly embarrassing as the person may be caught by surprise and unprepared. It also contributes to the woman reconsidering her next

overnight visit in an effort to avoid another occurrence.

Treatment Options
1. Behavioral Therapy

Behavioral therapy can help many types of functional incontinence. It is helpful to work with a physical therapist or occupational therapist to reduce barriers in getting to the bathroom, develop leg strength and gait, have a well-lighted bath with safety hand bars, wear comfortable and easy to remove clothing, do pelvic floor muscle exercises with biofeedback, practice urge suppression, and follow good fluid and diet habits.

2. Medications

Medications are not used specifically for this type of incontinence but may be used to relieve symptoms that become functional barriers, such as pain from arthritis.

3. Surgery

Surgery is not typically used to treat this incontinence. However, it can be used to eliminate the barrier, i.e., repair a bad knee or a broken hip.

Motivation and Compliance

Many of the treatment options for stress, urge, mixed, overflow and functional incontinence require behavioral changes. Behavioral techniques can be done every day within the framework of your lifestyle. They are things that you can explore and learn to do yourself. Like any type of behavioral change involving a habit or an exercise, motivation and compliance are a must. How do you get started?

There are many excellent books on fitness and exercise that address getting started and staying motivated. One that I especially like at my age is *Fitness after 50*[6] This book is written from the standpoint of not so much being able to run a marathon, but more with the goal of being fit enough to enjoy life and prevent problems. Craig Cuddeback, Co-director of Beverly Cracom Publications, stated

*"Daily exercise is like compounded interest on sav-
ings and investments. The more regularly you contribute to an active life-style, the greater the health
benefits. Being physically active is a small price to
pay for a healthy, productive future."* As I would say,
the more regularly you exercise your pelvic floor
muscles, the greater the benefits of bladder control
and pelvic floor support.[6]

The time spent strengthening this group of muscles is a small
price to pay for the great improvement in quality of life.

Another helpful book is slightly older, but has a primary focus
on motivation to continue your exercise program. It is called *Fitness
Motivation*[7]. It is written to prevent participant dropout from a fitness program and is quite appropriate for bladder fitness.

> *Compliance is preceded by awareness
> of the problem (ie wet clothing),
> education about the solution (seeing
> your healthcare giver, reading about
> the problem, talking to professionals,
> researching information), and
> motivation to succeed (wanting to be
> in control of your bladder again).*

Compliance to a behavioral program begins with the "need to
know". Very few people who are not directly affected by urinary
incontinence (self, friend, loved one) really care enough to learn about
urinary incontinence. Can you imagine trying to impress upon a 16-
year-old cheerleader the need to perform pelvic muscle exercises at
this time in her life, to avoid having bladder control problems later?
Only if she already had symptoms of urinary frequency or leakage
would she be inclined to practice pelvic floor muscle exercises. Talk
to her again after her first or second child, then she has a "need" to
know. But you can believe, the woman who has just had a baby and
now finds herself leaking urine, is ready to learn. She is ready to
commit to a program. Motivation has arrived. The need to know
comes with the problem.

> *The strongest motivator for compliance is your value for the outcome and your ability to see progress.*

Visual aids, audio aids, and biofeedback used with behavioral programs have been shown to be effective in encouraging motivation and compliance. Some of the organizations mentioned in the resource section of this book provide audio and video tapes. The use of diaries and telephone-linked care may also help. Perhaps the strongest motivator for compliance is your need to succeed and your ability to see progress. How much do you value the ability to control your bladder, the freedom from embarrassment, the confidence to take a trip, the security of lifting your child or grandchild without the loss of bladder control? Partnering with your physician or clinician, you can make a difference in your outcomes. This is where your motivation comes from, the value you put on the outcomes.

Behavioral changes are not easy to make. It may be difficult to give up a second cup of coffee, drink 8 glasses of water, do pelvic muscle exercises twice a day, or practice urge suppression techniques. However, being incontinent is not easy. This you already know. You can spend time, energy, and frustration in searching out toilets, changing clothing, providing excuses, and dealing with the emotional stress and feeling of embarrassment. Or, you can become proactive and determined to make your bladder life better. Habits are not easy to learn. But think of those that you already perform for your health and hygiene, brushing your teeth, taking a bath or shower, cutting your nails, moisturizing your face, washing your hands, shampooing your hair. How long does a shower take? Five minutes? More? Yes, these events take time, but you do them for yourself, because you value them. You may think brushing your teeth is a "bother" every morning, but you "know the need" so you routinely perform

the exercise. You don't want to experience bad breath, tooth decay, gum disease and loss of teeth. Think of pelvic floor muscle exercises in the same manner. You do not want to experience the shame and embarrassment, the odor, and the cost of urinary incontinence.

> *I have found that women with bladder control problems are very motivated to improve their symptoms. Some have dealt with embarrassing accidents, inconvenient pads, and even costly surgeries. Most are quite willing to be diligent with behavioral changes. ~DBS*

Social influences have an effect on behavior. This is seen in the exercise world where many people exercise in groups, have a running partner, or participate in community competitive races. Behavioral programs for incontinence are rarely done in social groups, but the social influence is still apparent in the outcomes. Urinary incontinence is not socially acceptable for adults. Use these influences, not for their negatives, but for their positives to help you remain committed. If you think a support group will help you, connect with one of the resources in Chapter 6 (NAFC) for contacts, newsletters and internet web sites. Make the most of social influence in your behavioral program.

Commitment to behavior changes will fluctuate as your daily responsibilities and priorities change. This is normal. If you do not follow through on your activities every day, do not consider yourself a failure. Urinary continence may not be your priority every day. If you do get away from your schedule, go back and review your reasons for wanting to participate in a behavioral program. In exercise fitness programs, this may be called a decision balance sheet. You weigh the benefits against the costs. Yours may look something like the following:

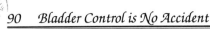

Decision Balance Sheet

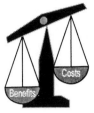

Benefits	**Costs**
Fewer leaks	Give up coffee
Less fear of embarrassment	Drink a lot of water
Don't always have to know where toilet is	Do my pelvic muscle exercises
Get to sleep at night	Practice urge suppression
Save money on pads	Try to lose weight
Feel more confident	Adds to my busy schedule
Get more work done	
Feel I have gained control	
Avoided surgery	
Helped myself	
Time for myself	
Less time tending to my incontinence	
Less chance for fall when I rush to the bathroom	
Less risk for bladder infections	
Don't have to worry about odor	
Can exercise without fear of leaks	

Make your own Decision Balance Sheet on the following form. Be honest with your benefits and costs. You may need to come back to it from time to time to re-evaluate your goals and commitment.

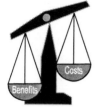

Date:_____

My Decision Balance Sheet

Benefits   *Costs*

_____   _____

_____   _____

_____   _____

_____   _____

_____   _____

_____   _____

_____   _____

_____   _____

_____   _____

Set goals to help remain focused and committed. A significant factor in attrition is disappointment in progress. With any muscle fitness program, progress requires considerable time and effort. Make short-term goals Evaluate your goals and progress periodically. You would not be able to run a marathon within the first month you decide to make that your goal. You would start with short-term goals, i.e. run two miles a day or run 14 miles a week; them build on those during the weeks that you train. Your overall goal of running 26 miles may be 10 months away. Set your continence goals similarly, starting where you are. If you are leaking 6 to 8 times day, perhaps your short-term goal would be to cut your leaks down to 5 times a day. Include some behaviors in your goals, such as drinking 5 glasses of water a day, trying to wait 10 minutes after an urge to urinate, cutting down to only one soda a day, or whatever might be appropriate for your situation. If you are getting up 5 times a night to urinate, start with a goal of only getting up 4 times a night. Make your goals short-term and realistic and specific. Reaching a goal provides positive feedback and encouragement. Long-term goals do have real value, but initially they can be overwhelming. View goal setting as steps-individually each is attainable.

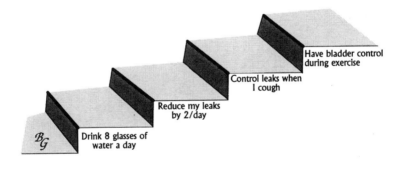

Quiz - Did you get it?

Match the types of incontinence with a descriptor

1. ___ Urge
2. ___ Overflow
3. ___ Functional
4. ___ Stress
5. ___ Reflex
6. ___ Mixed

a. leak urine when cough or sneeze
b. person with spinal cord injury
c. go to the bathroom frequently
d. can be caused by a urethral stricture
e. combination of stress and urge
f. something prevents access to toilet

Correct answers
1-c, 2-d, 3-f, 4-a, 5-b, 6-e

Myths-How are you doing so far?

Myth or Fact   (circle true or false)

True   False   1. Incontinence is a normal part of aging.

True   False   2. More women than men have symptoms
of incontinence.

True   False   3. Pregnancy and childbirth increase the
risk of incontinence.

True   False   4. Medications can contribute to incontinence.

True   False   5. After menopause, a woman cannot get
help for incontinence.

Correct answers   1 - False, 2 - True, 3 - True, 4 - True, 5 - False

ଈୠ *Chapter 3* ଔଷ

Self-Discovery

Self-Discovery

The information in this section will not only help you identify some of your own risk factors for incontinence, but will quantify the number of leaks and voids per day that you are now having, as well as the severity impact. This will give you a comparison for after you have implemented some behavioral techniques.

Personal Health Background
What are your risk factors?

Check the following risk factors that apply to you:
Female
_____ childbirth (how many _____)
_____ hysterectomy
_____ menopause
_____ previous radiation therapy to the pelvis

General
_____ age (over 50)
_____ overweight
_____ smoker
_____ partake in high impact exercises or exertion
_____ high caffeine intake (coffee, tea, soda, chocolate)

Following Conditions

____ stroke

____ Parkinson's

____ diabetes

Are there any of the above risk factors that you can control? Highlight those.

> NOTE: *Be sure to share this information with your healthcare provider for a specific and overall assessment and treatment plan. This does not take the place of an assessment by your healthcare provider, but is information that can be given to your provider to assist him/her in your diagnosis and treatment plan. This book is designed to provide general information and practical suggestions to help you become a more active participant in dealing with your symptoms. ~DBS*

Self Assessment

Medical History

a) Diabetes, stroke, Parkinson's, arthritis, lower back injury (indicate which)

b) Radiation therapy to pelvic area

c) Birth defect, type _____

Mobility

a) Need assistance getting to bathroom (i.e. cane, walker, another person etc.)

b) Need assistance getting clothing up

c) Have fallen within the past year with attempt to get to the bathroom.

Bowel Habits

Frequency

a) Once or more per day

b) Every 2-3 days

c) Every 4 or more days

Characteristics
a) Must strain to have bowel movement
b) Must use assistance to have bowel movement (enema, suppository, laxative)

Urinary Symptoms
a) Blood in urine
b) Pain or burning with urination
c) Strong or foul odor of urine
d) Difficulty in starting to urinate

Frequency of Urine Leaks
a) Once per day
b) 2-3 times per day
c) More than 3 times per day
d) Only at night
e) Number of times to bathroom per night_____

Activities Related to Urine Leaks
a) Coughing, laughing, sneezing, lifting
b) Exercising (jogging, aerobics, etc.)
c) Transferring from chair, getting out of bed, standing
d) On the way to toilet
e) Sexual intercourse

Onset of Urinary Leakage
a) After hysterectomy
b) After childbirth
c) Within past 6 months
d) Within past 2 years
e) Over 2 years

Amount of Urine Leaked
a) A little, minimal
b) A moderate amount
c) A large amount

Bladder Habits

Complete with the time you went to the bathroom, time you leaked, amount and time of fluid intake.

Date_____

Time	Void	Urine Leak Yes/No	Pad Change Yes/No	Fluid Intake*	Comments**
12 a.m.					
1 a.m.					
2 a.m.					
3 a.m.					
4 a.m.					
5 a.m.					
6 a.m.					
7 a.m.					
8 a.m.					
9 a.m.					
10 a.m.					
11 a.m.					
12 p.m.					
1 p.m.					
2 p.m.					
3 p.m.					
4 p.m.					
5 p.m.					
6 p.m.					
7 p.m.					
8 p.m.					
9 p.m.					
10 p.m.					
11 p.m.					

*Amount and type (i.e. 1 cup of coffee). **Did you leak a small or large amount, was your pad wet, did you leak on the way to the bathroom or before. What were you doing at the time (sneezing, exercising, having sex, lifting, etc.)

Complete the 24/hour bladder habit sheet then fill in the following:

1. How many times a day (24-hour) did I leak urine?_____

2. How many times a day did I go to the toilet a day? Add leaks + number of times urinated for total _____

3. How many times did I get up to go to the bathroom at night?
   _____

4. What was the average length of time between my voids?

5. How much fluid did I drink, in ounces. 8 oz = 1 cup, 10 oz = 1 glass.

6. Circle any of the following that you may have had in the 24 hours and the amount in ounces or number.

	Amount
Coffee	_____
Cola	_____
Citrus fruit juice	_____
Citrus fruit	_____
Chocolate	_____
Alcohol	_____
Artificial sweetener	_____
Spicy foods	_____
Tomato or tomato juice	_____

How Do I Manage My Symptoms?
Pads, tissue, towels, adult diapers, tampon, catheter, devices, scheduled toileting, medications. If you use pads or devices list type and number per day:_____

Skin Care Used for Incontinence
a) Soap
b) Moisturizer
c) Wipes

How do I rate the impact and severity of my symptoms on my life?
Complete the stress and urge incontinence severity indices.

Stress Incontinence Severity Index

Circle the appropriate number   Date_____

	Less than half the time	More than half the time
Over the past month how often have you leaked urine while laughing, coughing, lifting, sneezing, having sexual intercourse, or exercising?	1	3
Over the past month when you have leaked urine is it a:		
Few drops	1	3
Moderate amount	4	6
Large amount	7	9
Does urinary leakage affect any of the following for you?		
Work	1	3
Travel	1	3
Social activities	1	3
Exercise	1	3
Sexual activity	1	3

Total Points _____

Symptoms: Mild = 0-10 Moderate = 11-21 Severe = 22-27

Self-Rating Scale
On a scale of 1 to 10 (with 10 being the worst) how do you rate the severity of your incontinence at this time?   1 2 3 4 5 6 7 8 9 10

Urge Incontinence Severity Index

Circle the appropriate   Date_____

	Less than half the time	More than half the time
Over the past month how often have you had the urge to urinate yet leaked urine before reaching the toilet?	1	3
Over the past month how often do you have to get up at night to urinate?		
1 time	1	3
2-3 times	4	6
more than 3 times	7	9
Over the past month have you had to urinate more than once in a 2 hr. period?	1	3
Does urinary leakage affect any of the following for you?		
Work	1	3
Travel	1	3
Social activities	1	3
Exercise	1	3
Sexual activity	1	3

Total Points _____

Symptoms: Mild = 0-10 Moderate = 11-22 Severe = 23-30

Self-Rating Scale
On a scale of 1 to 10 (with 10
being the worst) how do you   1 2 3 4 5 6 7 8 9 10
rate the severity of your
incontinence at this time?

Fill in your number for your stress symptom index _____
Fill in your number for your urge symptom index _____

If you have three or more points on the stress incontinence severity index, consider that you have symptoms of stress incontinence. Up to 10 points may be considered mild, up to 21 points may be considered moderate incontinence.

If you have three or more points on the urge incontinence severity index, consider that you have symptoms of urge incontinence. Up to 10 points would be mild, up to 22 would be moderate, anything over 22 would be severe.

If you have three or more points on the urge scale and on the stress scale, consider that you have symptoms of mixed incontinence. Identify the behavioral treatments that are effective for both stress and urge symptoms.

These numbers are arbitrary. I personally consider three points on either scale severe, any urinary leakage or frequency is considered severe in my mind. The severity scale is just a point scale so you can keep track of the numbers. The real importance is how bothersome the problem is in your life.

> *Note: I have been intrigued by how low women rate the severity of their symptoms compared to how high men rate the severity of the same symptoms. Be open and honest with yourself about how disruptive your symptoms are to your everyday activities. ~DBS*

ɞ *Chapter 4* ଔ

Special Problems

Special Problems

Pelvic Floor Weakness

This is also known as pelvic floor relaxation.

Review: remember the description of the pelvic floor as a hammock of muscles or as a floor of support for a house. The muscles support the pelvic organs (uterus, bladder, urethra, and rectum). The muscles of the floor are held in place, connected to the bones of the pelvis by ligaments. Muscles stretch and contract. Ligaments have a finite amount of give or stretch beyond which they start to lose their elasticity.

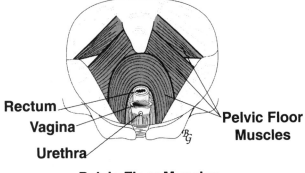

Rectum
Vagina
Urethra
Pelvic Floor Muscles

Pelvic Floor Muscles

Some of the surgical procedures for urinary incontinence in women consist of taking up the slack of these stretched tissues, lifting the muscle floor and providing support for the bladder. This helps until the ligaments are stretched again.

Pelvic floor weakness or relaxation can occur after pregnancy or childbirth, with obesity, with chronic straining for bowel movement, or with repeated exertion. To point out how amazing the pelvic floor is, think of what the female pelvic floor must accommodate, passages for urine and stool elimination, sexual intercourse, and childbirth. A tear or episiotomy with childbirth or a vaginal hysterectomy can be additional stressful events for the pelvic floor. Ligaments, muscles, blood vessels and nerves that pass through the muscles can be stretched or injured. Increasing pelvic muscle strength can help alleviate some of the symptoms associated with mild or moderate pelvic floor relaxation. Increasing muscle strength may reduce some of the stretching or strain on the muscles. More severe cases of pelvic relaxation may require surgical repair or pelvic support devices.

A note for the young, or not-so-young, active female. First, congratulations on your efforts to be active and fit. Do not view the need for pelvic floor muscle exercises as a negative. View it in the same manner as you would other components of fitness. For example, you may want your abdominal muscles to be strong and fit, not only for appearance, but for function (back support, ability to lift). However, the abdominal muscles, when they contract, create a force down against the bladder. This is why many women leak urine when they laugh, cough, sneeze, lift, or stand. The abdominal muscles contract, putting a force on the bladder that the closing sphincter and pelvic floor muscles may not be able to counter.

The pelvic ligaments and muscles of females with very active athletic lifestyles such as cheerleaders, gymnasts, tennis players, kickboxers, ballplayers, joggers, female paratroopers or hikers carrying a 40 pound backpack have a great deal of stress placed on them. The increased weight or impact of a jump in these activities compounds the force of gravity on the pelvic and abdominal organs, causing stretch and strain of the muscles and ligaments of the pelvic floor. Standing all day or being overweight also puts additional strain on the muscles of the pelvic floor.

Estrogen, the female hormone that diminishes with menopause, is important for vaginal and urethral tissue thickness and strength. It is also being studied for its role in ligament strength. For example, it is believed that women are more at risk for knee ligament injury during certain times in their menstrual cycle as estrogen fluctuates. Pelvic floor ligament injury in female paratroopers in the military is also being studied in relationship to menstrual cycle and estrogen levels.

If you are involved in exercise and fitness, learn how you can strengthen the group of muscles that make up the pelvic floor (pelvic floor muscle exercises). Add this group of muscles to your lifetime fitness plan. Start strengthening your pelvic floor muscles now if you want to minimize pelvic floor relaxation and avoid being the one out of four women who have urinary leakage. The risk factors are stacked against you if you are a woman.

Treatment Options
1. Behavioral techniques
Behavioral options for pelvic floor weakness include the following:
- Bladder training for urinary control
- Pelvic muscle exercises to develop strength and tone and provide support for the pelvic organs, increase urethral closing pressure and urinary continence
- Biofeedback to insure correct muscle contractions and measure the strength and endurance of those muscles
- Lifestyle and dietary modifications to reduce risk factors such as weight control and smoking cessation
- Education to avoid excess stresses on the pelvic floor and prevention of further progression by avoiding straining at stool, heavy lifting, standing up all day, and high impact exercise

2. Pelvic Support Devices
As a result of pelvic floor relaxation in women, some of the pelvic organs can protrude or herniate into the vagina. For example, the uterus can sag or drop down into the vagina. This is known as a *prolapse*. The bladder can push or bulge into the vaginal wall, similar to a hernia. This is known as a *cystocele*. A bulging of the rectum into the vaginal wall is known as a *rectocele*.

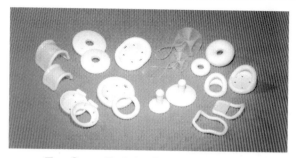

EvaCare Pelvic Support Devices
Courtesy of Mentor Corporation
Santa Barbara, CA

Some people with pelvic floor relaxation describe it as a feeling of heaviness in the pelvic region or complain of back pain. They may have difficulty with their walking exercise, and express a feeling similar to a "drag". The discomfort can be disabling.

Sheri is a 54 year-old mother of two. She has had a feeling of pelvic discomfort for some time. She describes it as like a "falling out" of her "bottom". She can actually see "something" coming from her vagina when she stands and uses a mirror to look between her legs. The problem is severe enough to interfere with her daily exercise walk. Sheri cares for an elderly parent with Alzheimer's Disease. She wants to avoid having surgery for the present time. Her doctor examined her and fitted her with a pelvic support device (pessary). 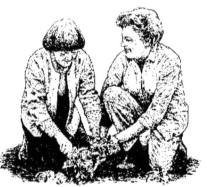 The pessary helped with the symptoms of discomfort and feeling of "falling out". It gave Sheri a way to manage her symptoms and problem of pelvic floor relaxation without surgery.

Pelvic support devices, or pessaries, can be inserted in the vagina to provide support for the vaginal walls or uterus. These support devices come in a variety of shapes and sizes depending upon the need of the person. They fill space in the vagina that is normally an empty space. They can provide support to the front of the vagina, back

of the vagina, top of the vagina, or all three areas. They are fitted by a physician or nurse practitioner. Once properly fitted, the pelvic support device should not be uncomfortable or interfere with urination or bowel movements. The patient usually is not aware of any sensation from the device. Some persons wearing pelvic support devices remove and clean their own device; others return to their healthcare provider to have the device removed and cleaned. Either way, the person using a pelvic support device must have follow-up exams and care to examine for proper fit, tissue irritation, and effectiveness of the device.

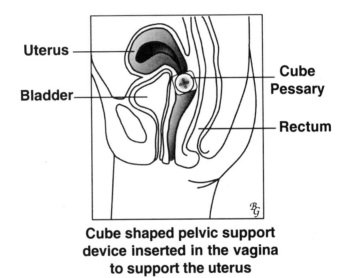

Uterus

Bladder

Cube Pessary

Rectum

Cube shaped pelvic support device inserted in the vagina to support the uterus

If you are using a pelvic support device, notify your doctor if you experience any of the following:
- Discomfort
- Pessary falls out
- Change in vaginal discharge
- Problems with urinating or bowel movement

Some women with pelvic floor relaxation wear a pelvic support device while waiting for a surgical procedure. Some wear a device in lieu of surgery. Discuss your individual situation and options with your healthcare provider.

Even if you do not have pelvic floor relaxation, committing to keeping your pelvic floor muscles strong will enable them to better withstand future stresses. The optimum situation would be to have this group of muscles strong and toned before cheerleading and sport activity days, before pregnancy and childbirth, before standing all day at work, before menopause. But even if your cheerleading and childbirth days are over, it is not too late to begin practicing pelvic floor health.

3. Surgery

There are a number of different surgical procedures for treating pelvic floor relaxation. Consult your physician regarding your options.

4. Medications

There are no medications specific for pelvic floor weakness, but estrogen replacement can help with tissue strength in post-menopausal women. Estrogen can be topically applied, (cream, suppository, ring) injected, taken orally or delivered via a skin patch. Ask your doctor or practitioner which is appropriate for you.

Exercise Incontinence

Some women experience bladder control problems only when they exercise. This is not uncommon. Up to one-third of women who do vigorous exercise will have some degree of urinary incontinence. ONE-THIRD!!!! Isn't it amazing this has not been addressed, for college athletes, for Olympians, for professional athletes???? What secrets we women can keep!!!!! Female athletes generally have well-developed abdominal muscles. However, very few will have had training in developing the muscles in their pelvic floor. The bladder and urethra may be in proper position during walking and non-exertion activities, but when the person participates in her specific sport or exercise, forces on the pelvic floor may allow urine to leak. The threshold needed to maintain continence is overcome during the physical stresses. Some may have an occasional

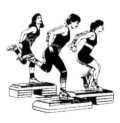

leak while playing tennis or while jumping on the trampoline with the children. Others may have routine urine leaks while jogging or doing aerobics. A study of female athletes at a major midwestern university showed that 28% of the females, average age 19.9 years, had urine loss while participating in their sport. Forty percent of these women first noted urinary leakage problems while in high school, and 17% first noticed problems while in junior high! These women were all elite, physically fit, college varsity athletes who had not experienced pregnancy and childbirth. Their major risk factor for urinary leakage was exercise. Not everyone that has a bladder control problem is an overweight older mother of several children. The sports associated with the most severe bladder control problems, in descending order, were gymnastics (67%), basketball (66%), tennis (50%), field hockey, track, swimming, volleyball, softball and golf.[8]

Review: The pelvic floor muscles are very important for providing support to the bladder and urethra. Remember the importance of the angle between the bladder and urethra to continence control. Contraction of the abdominal muscles sends a force down to the bladder and urethra. Extra support from the pelvic floor muscles can help the sphincters close tightly and prevent leakage.

Treatment options

There are several ways to prevent exercise incontinence. These approaches may be used together. The first is the fitness and/or preventive approach of developing strength in the pelvic floor muscles. This can help minimize pelvic floor relaxation and the slight drop of the bladder. Or, if you already are experiencing exercise incontinence, strengthening the muscles can help correct some degree of relaxation. This should be done for either minimizing or correction of an existing problem.

A second approach is the use of a pelvic floor support device while exercising. This can be as simple as a tampon or pelvic support device inserted in the vagina during exercise-enough to give support to the urethra for closing. The pessary may be used only with exercise; a sport pessary that can be inserted during activity, removed,

washed (or discarded if disposable), and stored until the next activity.

A third option is surgical correction of the pelvic floor relaxation as mentioned under stress incontinence. If this is chosen, pelvic floor muscle exercises should be performed after recovery from surgery so the muscles can continue to provide support.

Incontinence During Pregnancy and After Childbirth

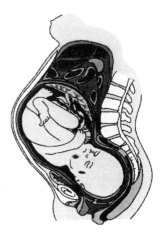

Women, as childbearers, have stresses on their pelvic floor that men never experience. That may be why at least two-thirds of all urinary incontinence cases are found in women. One of the most remarkable wonders of the female body is its ability to carry and deliver a newborn infant. The fact that a pear-sized organ, the uterus, can expand enough to house and feed a 7-pound baby, or two 5-pound babies, or even more, is a physiological feat. The tissues of the uterus, the blood vessels, the nerves and the muscles must stretch to accommodate the changes required for pregnancy and delivery.

Pregnancy and vaginal delivery are two major risk factors for female urinary incontinence. Although women who have not been pregnant can have incontinence, risk factors increase with pregnancy. It is the function of the pelvic floor, a structure of muscles and ligaments, to support organs of the pelvis. This includes the uterus, bladder, urethra and rectum. Proper support of these organs is important for control of urine elimination. Ligaments attach the muscles to the pelvic bones. Ligaments can stretch to a point, but then lose elasticity, tear or both. Muscles have more stretch capability than do ligaments. The nerves and blood vessels that run through the pelvic floor also have some stretch capability. During pregnancy, as the baby's weight increases, the forces upon the pelvic floor increase. As the uterus enlarges, the bladder is displaced. A pregnant woman often feels a need to go the bathroom more frequently because her bladder

does not have as much room in the pelvis to expand. She may also leak a little urine when she coughs, laughs, sneezes or lifts an object. This is called stress incontinence. The force of the abdomen contracting with the cough or sneeze overcomes the bladder sphincter or valve, causing some leakage.

As the baby grows, the pelvic floor must accommodate the increase in weight against gravity. The muscles and ligaments stretch. If the child is delivered vaginally, rather than by caesarian section, the opening has to stretch wide enough to allow the child's head to pass. The bladder, rectum, nerves and blood vessels are compressed against the pelvic bones. A large child, or prolonged labor, can cause the ligaments to tear slightly and nerves to be injured by the stretch. This can lead to a relaxation of the pelvic floor and a loss of support for the bladder, uterus and urethra. The risk of injury increases with each subsequent pregnancy and vaginal delivery.

Many women who have difficulty controlling their bladders during pregnancy recover shortly after delivery. However, with each subsequent pregnancy, recovery may take longer or may not be complete. A young mother may find that she leaks urine when she picks up her 6-month-old child, a symptom of stress incontinence.

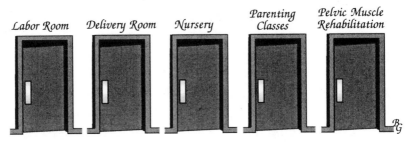

Women's Hospital
One Stop Delivery

Labor Room   Delivery Room   Nursery   Parenting Classes   Pelvic Muscle Rehabilitation

Things You Can Do

There are many variables that can affect the status of the pelvic floor after delivery: the difficulty and length of labor, the size and position of the infant, the size of the mother's pelvis, episiotomy, the number of children, the availability of medical care. Each person and each delivery is unique. The following suggestions may be helpful.

Before Pregnancy

If you have already had your child and are experiencing urinary leakage, prevention is too late for you. But it is not too late to minimize your incontinence risks with subsequent pregnancies. Pelvic muscle exercise is a technique for strengthening the support of the pelvic floor. Having your pelvic floor muscles and ligaments conditioned and toned is important before getting pregnant. Athletes do not participate in their sport without getting their leg, back, shoulder and neck muscles conditioned and strong. That would be a foolish risk of injury. Why would a female submit her pelvic floor to the extreme stress of pregnancy and vaginal delivery without being in the best condition? It is an invitation for injury. Exercising the pelvic floor muscles by performing correct Kegel exercises can help reduce stretch injury to the pelvic muscles and subsequent incontinence. The exercises must be performed correctly and consistently to get the maximal benefit. Many women have thought they were doing Kegels, but because of incorrect contractions were not getting their muscles stronger.

Another measure to consider before pregnancy is avoiding dehydration. This leads to constipation and straining to have a bowel movement. Straining increases the pressure and force down on the pelvic floor. Eat plenty of fruits, vegetables and fiber, and drink 8 glasses of water a day. Fluids also keep the urine diluted which is less irritating to the bladder. Drink plenty of water and avoid coffee, tea, colas or other agents that can be bladder irritants. For some women these can cause symptoms of frequency and urgency.

During Pregnancy

During pregnancy, avoid excessive pressure on your pelvic muscles when possible. This means avoid lifting heavy objects and standing for long periods of time. Avoid constipation and straining while having a bowel movement. Rest with your feet up when possible. Perform pelvic muscle exercises daily.

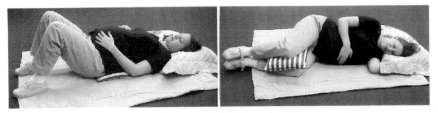

*Young pregnant woman doing pelvic muscle
exercises. Note positions and use of
pillows for comfort.*

After Pregnancy

After pregnancy, allow time for your pelvic floor muscles, ligaments, nerves and blood vessels to heal. Do not lift heavy objects, get off your feet when you can, avoid straining with bowel movement, and resume your pelvic muscle exercises.

Normally, the pelvic floor contracts by reflex of the nervous system. Immediately after childbirth, this reflex can be lost. If there has been significant pain, trauma, episiotomy, stitches or tearing during delivery, a reflex inhibition can occur. This is nature's way of protecting a swollen, injured or painful area. As healing occurs, teach your pelvic floor muscle to recover it's natural reflex action when coughing, sneezing, laughing or lifting. In other words, "brace" your muscle for the upcoming force.

Many women take a positive approach to returning their bodies to their pre-pregnant state. However, the pelvic floor is unseen and usually forgotten. The pelvic floor can suffer from fatigue as much as any other muscle in the body. A new mother needs rest for recovery.

Do not hesitate to discuss your symptoms with your doctor. Yes, it is very common to have urinary incontinence after childbirth. But do not accept it as a life long symptom.

Incontinence and Menopause

One of the exciting things about writing about menopause today is the freedom to discuss and write about this dynamic life process. Two hundred years ago, many women did not survive long enough to experience menopause. One hundred years ago, those women who did reach menopause were not allowed to mention it. Today, women

in large numbers are facing the changes that accompany menopause and actively looking for ways to remain in control.

Menopause refers to the cessation of ovarian function (production of estrogen) and menses (monthly period), the end of the reproductive years for a woman. *Note: it refers to the end of **repro-ductive** years, not **productive** years.* Today there are approximately 50 million women in the United States that have experienced menopause. Many women today can expect to live one-third of their life after menopause in a very productive manner.

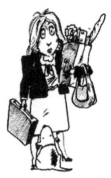

There are several health issues related to meno-pause that are widely known. They include bone loss (osteoporosis), hot flashes, mood swings, changes related to one's sex life, cardio-vascular risks and relationship to Alzheimer's Disease. Less publi-cized are the effects of menopause, or loss of estrogen, on a woman's urinary tract and pelvic floor. Although urinary incontinence can oc-cur at any age during a woman's life, many women notice that symp-toms begin or seem to worsen around this time in their life. Up to one fourth of women who have gone through menopause will experience urinary symptoms.

As menopause occurs, there is a drop in production of the hor-mone estrogen. The vaginal and urinary tissues in a woman are very sensitive to estrogen. Estrogen plays a role in the strength of the pel-vic floor muscles and ligaments and in the moisture of the vaginal and urethral tissues. For the urethra to close completely to prevent leak-age, it requires a certain degree of elasticity and moisture. Women may experience an increase in stress incontinence as well as an in-crease in bladder activity or urge incontinence with menopause. Es-trogen also affects the blood flow to the pelvic tissues, causing the lining of the vagina and urethra to be thinner, drier and more easily inflamed. Many women complain of vaginal dryness, itching, or irri-tation with menopause. Vaginal intercourse may become uncomfort-able because the tissues are drier and less elastic. Dr. Arthur Haney of Duke University describes the thickness of vaginal tissues before meno-pause as much like the area in the palm of the hand. After menopause, he describes the vaginal tissue thickness as somewhat like the back of

the hand. The urethral tissues may have similar changes and symptoms such as frequency, urgency, urinary tract infections or bladder leakage can occur.

Options

Women of menopause age today are for the large part healthy and active. They are concerned with health and fitness and quality of life. It is safe to say that for many quality of life includes bladder control and sexual health. Women are actively looking to healthcare practitioners to provide solutions.

The use of replacement estrogen, applied topically to the vagina (by cream, suppository, or pessary) is one option. Locally applied estrogen can help strengthen pelvic floor tissues, improve prolapse, and decrease irritative bladder symptoms (urgency and frequency). The tissues become thicker, more moist, and the urethra is able to close tighter, reducing the risk of urinary leakage.

If considering estrogen replacement therapy, discuss all of your options with your health practitioner. This applies even if you are considering "natural" or holistic estrogen sources. There are some situations in which supplemental estrogen should not be used. Generally women with breast, uterine, or cervical cancer or women with a history of blood clots or stroke may not be considered for systemic estrogen replacement. You need to know if systemic (by mouth, injection, or skin patch) or local applications (cream, suppository, pessary) are appropriate in your situation. There is no "one answer fits all" in regards to hormone replacement therapy. If you are not able to use estrogen replacement, there are vaginal moisturizers available over the counter. These can provide some relief for vaginal dryness and itching.

Pelvic Floor

If you are a person who has reached menopause with no thought to your pelvic floor, LISTEN UP! Your pelvic floor tissues will only get weaker with age. That means your risks for incontinence, prolapse (uterus drops), cystocele (bladder bulges in the vagina) and rectocele (rectum bulges in the vagina) increase. BUT, it is not too late. You can do a great deal to help yourself. Strengthening the pelvic

floor muscles with pelvic floor exercises and biofeedback, bladder training, weight loss (if needed) and hormone replacement therapy can all help to counter the effects that menopause has on the pelvic floor and bladder tissues. These behavioral therapies can also help to reduce the symptoms of stress and urge incontinence that are associated with menopause.

If you already have prolapse, you may not eliminate it, but you may be able to keep it from becoming worse by strengthening your pelvic floor muscles. Pelvic support devices (pessaries) can also be used to provide support and relieve symptoms of pelvic floor weakness. These devices can often offer sufficient support to decrease urinary incontinence.

Menopause is often a time when women begin taking a more active role in their health, supplementing vitamins, participating in exercise and fitness, incorporating a healthier diet, enjoying sexual activity and getting screening mammograms. It is a natural time to take an active role in pelvic floor health and continence.

If you happen to be reading this and are not yet in the menopause or perimenopause stage, the message is THE EARLIER, THE BETTER. Start now to get your pelvic floor muscles strong and toned. Do not be your mother's daughter with this (meaning do not wait until pelvic floor relaxation occurs to begin thinking about pelvic floor health). Include pelvic floor fitness in your lifestyle. Be more prepared than your mother was for menopause by doing your pelvic floor muscle exercises correctly and consistently. It is never too late to exercise and increase muscle strength. Practice weight management, adequate fluid intake, good bladder habits, and avoid lifting or exercises that increase forces on the pelvic floor.

Incontinence in the Workplace
Potty-gate and More

A few years ago incontinence in the "social" place made the news. A creative, bold (and perhaps even incontinent) young woman went in the male restroom at a NBA basketball game in Houston, Texas. Why? Because the line was shorter and she couldn't wait! I am not sure who complained, the women who did have to wait in the ladies line, or the men who were taken aback by her presence in the men's

room. But there was a complaint, followed by a counter complaint, regarding the lack of women's restroom facilities in public buildings.

Recently a small tourist town held a large event hosting thousands of tourists, the majority were female. The only complaint - not enough restrooms. Is this a surprise? Summertime, heat, fluids - what goes in must come out.

Why do such stories even make the news? And why does it seem mostly women who make the issue an issue. Is it so surprising that women who may have had a beer at a sports event would need to go to the bathroom? (Perhaps it was a surprise to the facility planners that women would be at a sports event). Yes, men have to go to the bathroom as well. But, one observation might be that their male anatomy and fly fronts make for much faster "down" time. Who says "life is fair"?

The Problem

Incontinence in the workplace is a very serious problem. This does not make the news and remains a silent, infrequently addressed issue for over a fifth of the women employed today. The consequences from incontinence in the workplace vary from embarrassment, increased urinary tract infections, quitting the job, to life-threatening self-dehydration in some of the more physically demanding careers.

Janice, a healthy and fit 38-year-old, was at work in her insurance office seeing a client. When she stood up to shake his hand, urine poured out on her skirt. In a face of panic, she picked up her brief case and purse, walked out, and never went back. Janice has become a recluse in her own home, pushing away family and friends. The experience devastated her. This is a severe but not isolated case. On a T.V. episode of NYPD Blue, officer Andy Sipowitz had an incontinent accident at work after his prostate surgery. His embarrassment and the reaction of his co-workers were openly shown to the audience. The message was clear; this is no laughing matter.

Today 59% of women are employed and most women in the workplace are fit and healthy. In a study of 1,113 white-collar female workers, 21% reported urinary incontinence. Blue collar female workers may have an even higher incidence because of increased risks for urinary incontinence from lifting, bending, standing, limited breaks and bathroom access. Laborers, mill workers, construction

workers, army recruits, nurses, physical therapists , any position requiring lifting, standing for long periods of time, or extended time
away from toilet facilities create added risk. Some women suffer
from urinary frequency and urgency, requiring frequent restroom breaks.
Some women who delay going to the bathroom for hours, such as
nurses and teachers, may develop bladder problems later in life.
"Holding" urine for hours on end can lead to an overstretched bladder, incomplete bladder emptying or frequent bladder infections.
Women may actually restrict their job opportunities because of limi-
tations placed on them with bladder control.

To deal with incontinence, women use containment pads, limit
fluids, avoid coffee and/or caffeine, frequently urinate and keep extra
clothes on hand to deal with the unpredictable event of urinary leakage while at work. Few women seek help from their physician or
nurse caregiver because of the ease of buying pads, low expectations
of help, the belief that incontinence was normal and the lack of information about help for the problem. But sadly to report, many who do
report their problem do not receive help. Their symptoms are dis-
missed by their healthcare provider and no solutions are offered. This
brings up the combination of two major concerns; 1) women need to
be more informed that there is help available as well as assertive in
seeking that help; 2)healthcare professionals need to be more informed
about the magnitude of effects incontinence can cause women in the
workplace and be prepared to initiate solutions.

The perception of urinary leakage as a social or hygienic problem is understandable. The embarrassment of an accident at work, at
a social event, or during sexual intercourse is enough to make some
women abstain from the activity rather than face the shame of someone knowing about their problem. Recent television ads for medication show men and women leaving the theater or sports events with
an urgent need to go to the bathroom. There are things that can be
done to help with the symptoms of urgency, frequency and urinary
leakage.

What Can You Do About It?

It is helpful to know what type of incontinence the symptoms rep-
resent. For example, women who leak urine when they laugh, cough,
sneeze, lift or exercise have symptoms of stress incontinence. Women

with symptoms of an urgent or frequent need to go to the bathroom have symptoms of urge incontinence. Many women have symptoms of both, which is known as mixed incontinence.

The following behavioral therapies can help improve bladder control:

For Stress Incontinence
- pelvic muscle rehabilitation (biofeedback and pelvic muscle therapy)
- dietary/fluid modifications
- weight control
- avoid constipation
- eliminate high impact exercise

For Urge Incontinence
- fluid management (decrease the intake of irritants, drink small amounts of water throughout the day, avoid becoming dehydrated)
- bladder training
- urge suppression
- scheduled voiding
- pelvic muscle exercises
- biofeedback

For Mixed Incontinence
- combination of the above suggestions

Know your rights in regards to bathroom access and frequency breaks. Educate yourself about the behavioral methods listed above and practice them. They can help reduce urinary symptoms in many incidences. Talk to your doctor or practitioner about appropriate therapy. Do not allow urinary incontinence to restrict your social or work life. Take control!

Incontinence During Sexual Activity

"From the first moment of conception, sexuality is an integral part of our being. It is genetically endowed, phenotypically embodied, hormonally nurtured, and matured by experience. The qualities of masculinity and femininity are inseparable from our personality. Our sexuality is manifested in our appearance, mannerisms, attitudes, and interpersonal relationships. It is ultimately expressed in our achievement of intimacy and gratification in our sexual encounters. Sexual function is both emotionally and physically the source of intense pleasure and gratification. It becomes, for each of us, precious, protected, privileged, and personal. The role sexual activity plays in our lives is as unique as our fingerprints, therefore, when a sexual problem occurs, the problem is unique for each person." — Dr. Andrew C. vonEshenbach, Urologist,[9] University of Texas M.D. Anderson Cancer Center, Houston, Texas and first Vice-President, American Cancer Society.

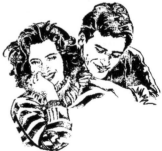

Urinary incontinence during sexual activity is a very personal and private issue that is rarely discussed. But, it occurs. It happens mostly in women who have symptoms of stress incontinence, meaning they leak urine with exertion or activity. It can also occur in women with symptoms of urge incontinence and it can occur in men, although less frequently than women. The activity of sexual intercourse as an exercise can cause urinary leakage from exertion and position changes. Urine can also leak from the bladder as the perineal muscles contract during orgasm or climax. Because you are probably blushing with embarrassment as you read this, let me frame this entire topic very matter-of-factly for you. Dr. vonEshenbach said it eloquently in his

quote. Being sexual is a normal part of one's life. Sex is not a dirty act, but can be a very special and intimate form of communication between two people who love each other. If there are problems with sexual activity, they can be discussed with healthcare practitioners. Rest assure, there are many other couples with this same problem.

Many health issues can affect sexual activity and intercourse. People with arthritis in their hips or back may find sexual activity difficult or certain positions painful. A variety of health problems (diabetes, vascular disease, stroke, depression) and/or medications can affect a woman's ability to find pleasure in sex. And many health conditions can affect one's own image and desire for sex. These health problems do not diminish the love between two people. But they may affect sexual activity, just as they may affect other parts of life. Because sexuality is an intimate form of communication and needs for intimacy are greater during illness or chronic health problems, it is important to address this situation and search for solutions.

> *Side bar: I had a patient a few years ago who had surgery to remove his urinary bladder because of cancer. In most instances, this surgery causes erectile dysfunction (impotence or the inability to have an erection). The gentleman commented "I guess my wife will not love me anymore!" A student nurse caring for him wisely responded " Did you make love to your wife every night?" He replied "no". The student said, "Did you love her any less on the nights that you did not make love to her?" I thought what she said was a very wise and insightful comment that gave the patient a chance to think about his relationship with his wife and offered reassurance that interpersonal love does not depend upon intercourse. ~ DBS*

Leakage of urine during sexual intercourse can occur during penetration or during orgasm. Incontinence during penetration is likely a "stress" type incontinence from the pressure of the penis on the back of the bladder wall or the bladder base. (Remember, the female bladder lies just in front of the vagina.) Usually, the woman would have

symptoms of stress incontinence at other times, such as when she laughs or coughs. Incontinence during orgasm is likely related to urge incontinence, where the bladder is provoked to instability by the orgasm. It is possible to help this type of incontinence by taking an "urge incontinence medication" a few hours before intercourse. That is, assuming intercourse is planned, which it frequently is not. Strengthening the pelvic floor muscles could help with the "stress type" incontinence of penetration. Not only would the pelvic muscle exercises help control the incontinence, but they may even enhance sexual enjoyment for the man and the woman. The use of a smaller pelvic support device may prevent leakage and still not interfere with intercourse.

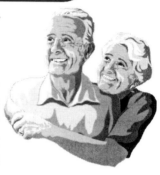

"They say you pick up speed when you get older."

I am sure you want to "fix" this problem. I encourage you to seek help from your doctor and to do exercises to strengthen your pelvic muscles. But, while you are addressing these possible solutions, let's explore these thoughts. Of course, urinary leakage during sexual activities does not sound very romantic. But, think about this. Urine is sterile when it comes out of the body. It is not dirty. It is cleaner than your mouth (kisses), and probably cleaner than your hands (caresses). So, even though not a first choice, a little urine will not hurt your partner. To minimize leakage, go to the toilet before sex play begins and attempt to double void and empty your bladder. If necessary, place a pad under you on the bed (or wherever) for protection of the linens. Having a washcloth nearby can provide you with a quick cleanup tool. I do not intend to make light of your symptoms, but would like to reassure you that this occurs with other couples. You are not the only one. Consider the problem of incontinence during sex as unfortunate, but manageable. The emotional expression and closeness of sexual activity are much more important than the physical aesthetics.

Communication is so important, yet most of us are very poor at communicating about private, personal health issues. Mixing urinary leakage and sex must be the ultimate private issue. This is where you

need to be brave. Do not suffer with this problem in silence. If you are having incontinence, explain to your partner that this is a problem you are having, that you wished you weren't, but that you do not want to give up sexual intimacy because of it. Ask him to be understanding and patient. Most partners, when they understand the situation, do not consider this to be a big deal. It usually bothers the one who is leaking more than the partner. After your sex play, perhaps just go take a shower together. Lighten up, do not make this issue "an end of the world" or tragic type issue. Urinary incontinence affects many people, young and old. Making excuses to avoid sexual activity will only leave your partner wondering if something is wrong, asking himself if he is less desirable or if you have stopped loving him.

Do not let incontinence control your life, seek isolation, or stop doing everyday activities. Be determined to continue those things in your life that interest you. Allowing urinary incontinence to force you to give up exercise, travel, social events, or sex is not healthy for you or your family. If you are a woman with the problem of urinary leakage during sex, and you are in a warm, loving, sexual relationship, communicate openly and problem-solve with your partner about this issue.

If you are the partner of a woman who has incontinence during sexual activity, be supportive. Keep a sense of humor, help with the hygiene part, and carry on with a matter-of-fact and loving attitude. Do not act offended or relate the incontinence to child-like behavior. This could potentially be demeaning or belittling to your partner. Any message from you that relays lack of acceptance will make your partner more reluctant to participate in sexual activity. As a partner, your acceptance is of great importance. Touching and sexual activity communicate acceptance.

> *Side bar: I had a patient who had stopped sleeping in the same bed with her husband because of her night-time frequency and sometimes bedwetting. His interpretation was that she did not love him anymore. When, in fact, she was doing it out of consideration for him. After he brought up his concerns to me, I guided them*

towards saying to each other what they had said in private to me. He wanted her closeness and was not willing to lose it because of her incontinence. ~DBS

Nocturia in Adults

Nocturia in adults refers to being awakened at night with the need to go to the bathroom. *Noct* is a prefix pertaining to the night, *uria* pertains to urination. Nocturia is a common clinical complaint of adults. Nocturia is the most age dependent of lower urinary tract symptoms and is frequently seen in otherwise "healthy" elderly women. For persons under the age of 65 it is considered normal to awaken once at night for the bathroom. For those over the age of 65 it is considered normal to have up to two episodes of going to the bathroom at night. Getting up at night more than twice is generally considered nocturia. It is not the same as nocturnal enuresis which refers to leaking urine during sleep.

It is important to distinguish if the nighttime events of going to the bathroom are true nocturia. True nocturia refers to being awakened because of the urge to go to the bathroom. The need to go to the bathroom is actually what awakens the person. It does not refer to the situation where a person is awakened by some other cause, such as pain, insomnia, or a noise disturbance and then, incidentally, goes to the bathroom. Repeatedly getting up to go the bathroom when awake for some other reason can eventually become a habit, causing the person to think she has to get up for the bathroom. Rarely, this occurs as a lifelong habit or the result of an anxious personality trait, with the person thinking she has to use every available opportunity to go to the bathroom.

Not only is nocturia annoying, but it can result in sleep deprivation, fatigue, and traumatic injury from falls while navigating to the bathroom at night. Often the symptom presented to the physician is daytime tiredness or insomnia. Urinary frequency with discomfort may indicate inflammation of the bladder. Urinary frequency without discomfort may indicate excessive fluid intake, diabetes, congestive heart failure or a medication effect.

Factors leading to nocturia can be singular or mixed. With nocturia, there are basic underlying factors: the volume of urine output

can increase during the night; the bladder capacity can diminish during hours of sleep; or a combination of the two. Forty-three percent of those with nocturia have an overproduction of urine at night. This is more common in the elderly. The circadian rhythm of the antidiuretic hormone may be altered affecting the amount of urine made at specific times of the 24-hour period; the filtration rate of the kidney may be decreased affecting how much fluid is conserved; or the cardiovascular system may not be able to pump enough blood to the kidneys during waking hours. When the latter occurs more blood goes to the kidneys during sleep, causing more urine to be made while at rest. Specific causes behind the nocturia can be cardiovascular disease, diabetes, lower urinary tract obstruction or urinary retention, stroke, peripheral edema, unstable bladder, diuretic medications taken near bedtime, caffeine, alcohol, or increased consumption of fluids at bedtime. Situations causing the bladder to be overactive and have a diminished capacity at nighttime can be anxiety, bladder stones, cancer of the bladder, urethra, cystitis, medications, or overactive bladder.

Evaluation

It is important to see your doctor or practitioner to establish the cause of nocturia. A focused history should be taken along with a physical examination. A 24/hour voiding diary can demonstrate how much urine is being excreted at night and provide an estimate of the capacity of the bladder. This can help categorize the nocturia as increased urine output, overactive bladder or a combination of the two. Fluid intake patterns, medications, past surgery and other disease conditions should be considered. Signs of diabetes and congestive heart failure should be particularly looked for. Diagnostic tests to look at function disorders of the bladder are also performed if necessary.

Treatment Options

Because bladder problems are not always the cause of nocturia, the treatment will only be effective if it is aimed at the cause. For example, if the cause is congestive heart failure and peripheral edema (fluid collecting in the legs), the treatment should address the congestive heart failure and the edema. Fluid management behaviors can be

helpful, such as taking more fluids in the morning and less in the afternoon, restricting fluids a few hours before bedtime. Restricting salt
intake can help reduce fluid retention. Diuretics may be given in the
middle to late afternoon, with the idea that they will take effect before
bedtime. Lying down for an hour or so before dinner, letting the fluid
that is built up in the legs return to circulation and the kidneys, and
then getting up to go to the bathroom helps to eliminate some of the
accumulated fluid. Applying compression hose or stockings first thing
in the morning can help minimize fluid build-up in the lower legs.

Dietary modification to avoid bladder irritants such as alcohol
and caffeine can be helpful to those who have nocturia due to an
irritative bladder. Bladder training through the day to train the bladder to hold more urine is appropriate for those who have an overactive bladder. Pelvic floor muscle strengthening is a part of the bladder training process. Gradually set goals of trying to increase time
between voids by 15 minute intervals to increase bladder capacity.
At nighttime try to resist the first urge and go back to sleep. With the
next urge, get up and go to the bathroom. Try to suppress the next
urge, and so on. For example, if getting up 4 or 5 times/night, try to
decrease it to 2 or 3, then 2 or 1.

Medications may be effective in treating nocturia. Use of an antidiuretic hormone is an option with adults. If this option is used, the
person must be monitored for symptoms such as headache or
lightheadedness which might suggest electrolyte depletion. Side effects are rare in children, but may occur in the elderly, especially those
with congestive heart failure. Anticholinergic medications may be
used in cases of bladder overactivity. These can be effective in inhibiting bladder contractility and in increasing the bladder capacity.

Because some people will have a mixture of causes, a combination of therapies might be appropriate to use. Evaluation by your
physician is needed to determine the most appropriate treatment options. The success of treatments can be evaluated with the use of the
24/hour bladder diary.

Quiz   Did you get it?

Match the following

_____1. Pelvic floor relaxation

a. uterus dropping down in the vagina

_____ 2. Exercise incontinence

b. more common in women because of vaginal opening

_____ 3. Bedwetting

c. nighttime urinary frequency

_____ 4. Prolapse

d. pelvic support device

_____ 5. Pessary

e. person leaking urine with exertion or activity

_____ 6. Nocturia

f. most common voiding problem in children

Correct Answers
1 - b, 2 - e, 3 - f, 4 - a, 5 - d, 6 - c

✳ Chapter 5 ✳

Continence Management Plans

Continence Management Plans

"Real People" Update

In the first section of the book we mentioned some real people who had bladder control problems? They all sought help and were treated. Here is the rest of their story.

*A*nn, a 34 year-old mother of three.

Problem: Ann leaked urine when she coughed, laughed, sneezed, picked up her child, or had sexual intercourse; she was up two or three times a night to go to the bathroom.

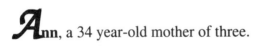

Goal: To reduce her number of day-time leaks and to decrease her waking times at night to go to the bathroom.

Events: For help, Ann was talking with a friend when the friend casually said, "don't make me laugh so hard, I will wet my pants". Ann replied "you, too?" She realized that she was not the only one with a bladder control problem as they talked and compared symptoms. On Ann's next visit to her doctor, she asked if losing bladder control was nor-

mal and if there were treatments.

Approach: A bladder history and assessment were taken by her doctor. Ann provided a three-day fluid/bladder habit sheet and she was checked for a urinary tract infection. Her doctor examined her and found a mild degree of pelvic floor relaxation and noted that when he asked her to cough or bear down, she leaked urine. He started her on a behavioral program for bladder control.

Ann started pelvic muscle exercises with a home biofeedback unit. She also reduced her coffee intake and increased her water intake. She practiced her exercises initially at home with her biofeedback trainer. Eventually she learned to perform a pelvic muscle contraction just before she would laugh, cough, sneeze or lift her child. By week four of her exercise program, Ann was beginning to see progress in her symptoms. By week 10 she was not getting up at all during the night for the bathroom. By week 14, she only had an occasional leak in the daytime versus the two or three times before she started her program. She no longer feels the need to wear a pad. An occasional leak "accident" is now a major event rather than an everyday occurrence. At the time of this writing, Ann is pregnant with her fourth child and continues her pelvic muscle exercise program. She realizes it will be a life-long effort for her.

Ann said, "I used to go to the bathroom nearly every hour or so until I started using urge suppression and scheduled toileting. Now I am not in the bathroom at every store and still don't have to get up at night, even though I am pregnant".

*M*ary, a 53 year-old nurse.

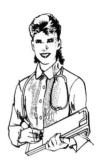

Problem: Mary leaked urine when she laughed, coughed or jogged and had a small amount of urine dribble when she stood up after using the toilet.

Goal: To not leak urine or have to wear a pad in her panties.

Events: Mary spoke with a continence nurse after attending a lecture on incontinence.

Approach: The nurse discussed behavioral options with Mary. Mary started practicing pelvic muscle exercises using home biofeedback. She practiced doing a quick pelvic floor muscle contraction as she started to cough or sneeze. After 8 weeks of exercising she had less leakage and was not dribbling as much. After 16 weeks she no longer leaked urine with exertion and stopped dribbling after she urinated.

Mary said, "Leaking urine was terrible for me. Now I can jog with confidence that I won't leak and not worry about being embarrassed when I laugh or cough".

*A*ngie, a 23 year-old single, competitive swimmer.

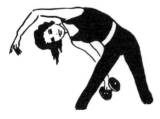

Problem: Angie had urge incontinence, voiding every hour or so during the day and getting up 4 to 5 times every night to void.

Goal: To not have to go to the bathroom so often.

Events: Since childhood, Angie had always had close physician contact regarding her symptoms. Her physician enrolled her as a participant in a pilot project to test a new home biofeedback unit.

Approach: Angie started home biofeedback and pelvic muscle exercises as part of a 16-week behavioral program. She also practiced bladder training, urge suppression and fluid management. She saw results very quickly by doing her pelvic floor muscle exercises five minutes, twice a day. By week four she was getting up less at night for the bathroom and voiding less frequently in the day. By week nine she was sleeping 8 hours without interruption and her voids in the daytime decreased from 11 to 8. Her overall voids in a 24/hour period decreased from 16 to 8.

Angie said, "I can go all night without interruption. To me, that's wonderful".

*A*unt Doris, a 76-year-old mother of 5 who lived in assisted living.

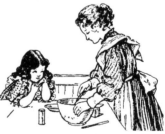

Problem: Doris leaked urine when she laughed, sneezed or coughed. She had difficulty getting to the bathroom and was becoming socially isolated.

Goal: To reduce her number of leaks and to assure that she would reach the bathroom safely, without leaking urine or falling.

Events: Doris began seeing a physical therapist (PT) for her Parkinson's disease. The PT become aware of her bladder control problem and started her on a continence program.

Approach: An assessment and 24-hour bladder/fluid diary were recorded for Doris. It was discovered that she leaked 8 to 10 times a day, that she knew when she needed to get to the toilet, but felt she could not get there in time. She was also drinking several cups of hot chocolate a day with artificial sweetener. She started pelvic muscle exercises, a toileting schedule, urge suppression, fluid management and strengthening exercises for her arms and legs. She began doing pelvic muscle exercises twice a day. She went to the bathroom upon waking, immediately after breakfast, mid-morning, after lunch, mid-afternoon, before dinner, after dinner, at bedtime, and once during the night.

She practiced urge suppression by taking a deep breath, relaxing, doing a pelvic muscle contraction, then slowly moving to the bathroom. She reduced her intake of cocoa and artificial sweeteners to one cup a day and began drinking more water throughout the day. The physical therapist worked with her on arm and leg exercises to improve her balance, strength, gait and mobility. An occupational therapist also worked with her to help select underwear and clothing that permitted easier access to the toilet. The therapist also introduced her to a more effective urinary pad that protected her clothing. Doris was quite motivated to follow her program and remain independent in assisted living, so she was compliant and consistent with her exercises and fluids. She decreased her leaks to a more manageable two or three a day and also felt more secure about her mobility. With appropriate continence undergarments, she no longer had to worry about odor or wet marks on her clothing.

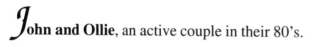

> *Doris said, "I was so afraid I would be sent to a nursing home. I did not want anyone to know about my problem. Sara, my PT, has been a Godsend for me. She has helped me so much. Now I can go out and visit my son and his family without being afraid of an accident."*

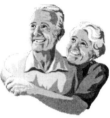

*J*ohn and Ollie, an active couple in their 80's.

They live in a retirement village.

Problem: Ollie had a problem with bladder control that was worse at night. She would get her clothing and the bed wet every night, waking John. Medications for this made her dizzy and she fell, breaking a hip.

Goal: To help Ollie get through the night without getting her clothing and bed wet.

Events: John and Ollie have spoken to several doctors about this problem. Attempts have been made to help her with medications, behavioral therapy, and fluid management. Although the medications helped her with her urinary symptoms, she could not tolerate the side effects of dizziness and they were discontinued.

Approach: Nighttime toileting (nocturia) or bedwetting is fairly common in older adults. Many people live with getting up 4 to 5 times a night to void. However, urinary leakage that is occurring 4 to 5 times a night is quite distressing. Sleep is disturbed, the partner is disturbed, and risks for falls increase. Hips are broken and heads are cracked. Ollie was examined for urinary tract infection, diabetes, heart disease and other conditions that may contribute to nocturia. She was asked about pain, a common finding in persons who awake frequently at night. A bladder/fluid diary was

kept. Her medications were reviewed to see if there were any contributing factors from them. The urologist also did bladder studies. The only conclusive finding was that her nighttime voiding volume was greater than her daytime fluid volume. John and Ollie were adamant about not taking any more medication after she fell and broke her hip. They already practiced evening fluid restriction and limiting of bladder irritants. She rested every afternoon with her feet elevated. Although these actions helped, they did not totally solve her night accidents. Because several treatment options had been tried without success, goals were changed to safely managing her nighttime incontinence without sleep disruption and to protect her skin. Ollie was shown cotton continence underwear for women with a super absorbent pad insert that could actually hold three voids and not feel wet against the skin. These are commonly used for patients with Alzheimer's Disease to let them sleep through the night. Waking people with Alzheimer's Disease often leaves them awake and roaming the rest of the night, disturbing others who are trying to sleep. With this continence system, plus a skin care product and a pad for the bed, Ollie and John were able to sleep through the night, even though she was "leaking" urine. Her clothing and bedding remained dry. While this was not the optimum choice for leakage, it was a reasonable choice for this couple, realizing how many treatments they had tried and their desire to get through the night safely and without interruptions.

Ollie said, "I am so grateful for everything you have done." John said "I have literally tried everything and still would have to change the sheets at least once every night. I was so tired. Thank you for telling us about these products".

In Review: Things I can Do

Management plans specific for the various types of incontinence symptoms are summarized for a quick referral in the following section. Refer to earlier text for more detailed information.

Stress Symptoms

WHO am I

- Women with children
- Women who exercise or do physical labor
- Women after menopause
- Women with a chronic cough
- Women who are overweight
- Women who chronically strain to have a bowel movement

WHAT do I have

- Symptoms of urinary leakage with laughing, coughing, sneezing, lifting, exercise, standing

HOW can I improve

- Keep a 24-hour bladder diary to record when you leak
- Begin a pelvic floor muscle exercise program (work on strength and endurance)
- Use home or office biofeedback
- Practice performing a pelvic muscle contraction just before you cough, laugh, sneeze, lift or stand
- Practice double voiding
- Lose weight if needed
- Stop smoking
- Manage constipation
- If past menopause, consider topical estrogen therapy
- Use a pelvic floor support device if recommended by doctor or practitioner

Urge Symptoms

WHO am I

- Women with irritative bladder symptoms
- Women with an overactive bladder
- Women who are pregnant
- Women who are past menopause

WHAT do I have

- Symptoms of frequency, urgency
- Have to get to bathroom in a hurry
- May go to toilet 15 to 20 times a day, with minimal leakage of urine
- May leak before getting to toilet
- Get up to go to the bathroom several times a night

HOW do I improve

- Keep a 24-hour bladder and fluid sheet
- Record when you leak in relation to what you drink
- Eliminate bladder irritants
- Drink 6 to 8 glasses of water a day (but not in large amounts at one time)
- Drink fluids throughout the day, rather than in 2 to 3 sittings
- Reduce fluid intake after evening meal
- Get bladder infections (if present) treated
- Practice pelvic muscle exercises
- Use home or in-office biofeedback
- Practice bladder training using urge suppression
- Stop smoking
- Provide a safe bathroom environment (lighting, handrails)
- If having problems with mobility, work on gait, balance and leg strength, BE safe
- Wear clothing that is easy to remove quickly

Mixed Symptoms

WHO am I

- Women with children

- Women who exercise or do physical labor
- Women after menopause
- Women with irritative bladder symptoms
- Women with overactive bladder

WHAT do I have
- Leak urine when cough, laugh, sneeze, exercise, lift, stand
- Have to urinate frequently
- Must reach toilet in a hurry
- Get up at night for the bathroom more than once
- Feel strong, almost painful, urge to void

HOW do I improve
- Keep a 24-hour bladder/fluid diary
- Identify fluids or foods that increase urge
- Avoid fluids or foods that make your bladder more active
- Begin a pelvic floor muscle exercise program
- Do home or office biofeedback
- Do bladder training with urge suppression to increase bladder capacity
- Drink 6 to 8 glasses of water a day (but not in large amounts at once)
- Drink fluids in small amounts throughout the day, rather than at two or three sittings
- Practice pelvic muscle contraction before laugh, cough, sneeze, lift or stand
- Double void
- Lose weight if needed
- Stop smoking
- Provide a safe bathroom environment (lighting, handbars)
- Develop good gait, balance and lower limb strength to prevent falls (be safe)
- Wear clothing easily removed for toileting

Overflow Symptoms

WHO am I

- Women who have had bladder surgery
- Women who are pregnant
- Women with constipation
- Women with urethral stricture or urethral narrowing
- Women with spinal cord injury
- Women with diabetes

WHAT do I have

- Not able to get urine stream started
- Not able to fully empty bladder
- Go to the bathroom, void a small amount then have to return again in a few minutes
- Leak small amounts of urine as bladder overflows

HOW do I improve

- See your doctor for evaluation
- Practice double voiding
- Change positions while urinating
- Press down on your bladder with your hand while trying to urinate
- Do not wait long periods of time (i.e. over 4 to 5 hours) before trying to urinate in the daytime (you don't want your bladder to overfill or bladder muscle to overstretch)

Bedwetting Symptoms

WHO am I

- Children between ages of 5 and 16 who wet the bed more than twice a month

WHAT do I have

- Not able to wake up at night to go to the toilet

HOW do I improve

- Get an evaluation to rule out medical problems

- If the child is old enough and willing, begin a behavioral program
- Be careful not to reflect shame, embarrassment, disappointment or punishment
- Work with behavioral techniques appropriate to and interesting to the age and likes of the child (incorporate sports, music, art, movies, etc)
- Practice behavioral approaches such as decreased fluid intake after dinner, urge suppression, pelvic muscle exercises

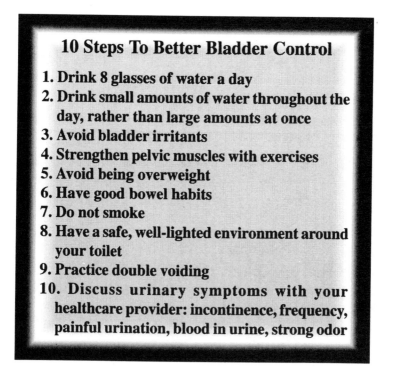

10 Steps To Better Bladder Control

1. Drink 8 glasses of water a day
2. Drink small amounts of water throughout the day, rather than large amounts at once
3. Avoid bladder irritants
4. Strengthen pelvic muscles with exercises
5. Avoid being overweight
6. Have good bowel habits
7. Do not smoke
8. Have a safe, well-lighted environment around your toilet
9. Practice double voiding
10. Discuss urinary symptoms with your healthcare provider: incontinence, frequency, painful urination, blood in urine, strong odor

Bedwetting in Children

Up to 10 million children are affected by urinary incontinence at night. This is commonly called bedwetting or sleepwetting. In medical terms it is called nocturnal (night) enuresis (leaking of urine) or sleep enuresis. It can be primary, referring to children who have never had nighttime control of urine, or secondary, referring to children who were dry for 6 to 12 months then lost control. Primary sleep enuresis is the most common type of bedwetting.

> *"I knew that bedwetting was a) wicked and b) out-side my control...It was therefore possible to sin without knowing you committed it, without wanting to commit it, and without being able to avoid it..."*
> *George Orwell, 1950,*
> *In Sheldon & Wacksman "Enuresis" In Urinary Incontinence*
> *-PD O'Donnell[10]*

Bedwetting is the most common voiding problem in children. It refers to children over the age of five that wet the bed more than twice monthly. Bedwetting affects 15% of children at age 5. Most children grow out of bedwetting. By age 7, the number drops to 10%; by age 10, 7% of children are bedwetters. This is a significant number of

children that are affected. The good news is that bedwetting does not reflect a serious medical condition in most children. The bad news is that bedwetting does affect the child's self-esteem, socialization, and the family's dynamics. It can trigger abusive relationships. Bedwetting becomes such a problem that 95% of the parents of children who are bedwetters seek professional help. Con-

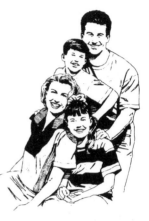

versely, only about 25% of adults with incontinence will seek help. Parents generally expect their child to be toilet trained earlier than physicians project. Bowel control is achieved on the average at 18 to 24 months; daytime bladder control at an average of 4 years; and nighttime bladder control at an average 4 1/2 . Each child is different and these are just averages, meaning some children will be younger and some will be older. But about 15% of children will still be wetting the bed at age 5.

The incidence of bedwetting does run in families. If one parent was a childhood bedwetter, the child has a 43% chance of being a bedwetter. If both parents were bedwetters, the incidence rises to 77% for the child. The occurrence is higher for boys than for girls. A small number of children who are bedwetters do have medical conditions that need to be explored. Kidney disease or abnormalities, urinary tract infections, and conditions such as diabetes need to be ruled out by your physician. Other possible causes of bedwetting are:

- Increase in the number of uninhibited bladder contractions
- Small bladder capacity
- Greater urine production
- Deeper sleep
- Constipation
- Food allergies
- Pinworms

These factors may interact as a cause and not be a single contributor. It is NOT believed that children wet the bed deliberately or that

Medications

Medications can be used to treat bedwetting. They may be used when behavioral therapies fail or in combination with behavioral options. Discuss this with your child's physician.

Combination Therapy

Quicker results may be seen when treatments are combined, such as medications, alarm, and behavioral therapies.

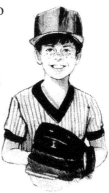

*R*andy is the seven-year-old second grader who is a bedwetter.

Problem: He still wets his bed at night, several times a week.

Goal: To get better control of his nighttime bedwetting.

Event: His pediatrician was aware of this problem and at age seven a urologist was consulted. After some tests were done, a behavioral approach was recommended. The continence nurse began working with Randy and his mother.

Approach: Randy was very motivated to try and get better. He joined his mother in talking to the nurse. The nurse carefully explained to Randy that many children, especially boys had the same problem. She clearly mentioned that he was doing nothing wrong and should not feel ashamed or embarrassed. She also emphasized that the program they were discussing was not a punishment. It was to help him learn to train himself to wake up when he needed to urinate. She said the program would take time and patience, but that most children did improve.

Randy was agreeable to trying the program, even though it meant he would have to take more responsibility. His mother was very supportive and said she would help him but not take sole responsibility, he would have to be a partner and do his share.

Randy lived in Colorado and was a Colorado Rockies baseball fan. The program designed for him was set up similar to a baseball game for the purpose of keeping score or to document Randy's progress. The seven days of a week represented seven innings of a game. The program of 10 weeks represented 10 games. Randy represented the Rockies, the bed was known as the Bandits. A scoreboard was set up on a poster in Randy's room.

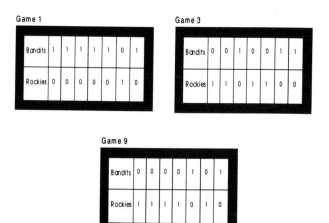

Each night if Randy stayed dry, he would get credit for a run for that inning of the game (week). If he wet his bed, the Bandits would get a run for the night (inning). Thus the score would go for the week, making up one game. If Randy did win the game (for the week), his mother and father would reward him with a special outing or a Rockies memento. At the end of the 10-week season, if he was

over 500 in his games there was another reward. Randy made his own scoreboard, and was responsible for keeping his own score. He was quite creative in designing his board, using Rockies baseball colors and putting up some of his baseball cards around the poster. It was his secret game, but he could proudly display it in his room without his friends knowing the actual meaning.

The ritual that Randy began to follow (he called the first week Spring Training, weeks 2-9 the Season, and week 10, the World Series) is as follows:

In the daytime, Randy worked to delay each void by 15 minutes (without an accident) in an effort to help his bladder stretch and hold more urine. After dinner, he restricted his fluid intake. He did not drink milk or any caffeine drinks or chocolate after 2pm in the afternoon. His bedtime reading was at 8pm, lights out at 8:30. Just before lights out, he went to the toilet, leaving a night light for the hall and bathroom. He left clean pajamas and bedding by his bed. He put a bed-wetting sensor in his underpants. This would alarm as soon as it was wet with urine, awakening Randy. When the alarm sounded, he was to practice doing a pelvic muscle contraction to stop his flow of urine, disconnect the sensor, and then slowly move to the toilet. Randy was told that it would probably take several nights for him to start responding to the alarm and being able to stop the flow of urine. He was not to get discouraged if he could not do it right away. For the first 3 to 4 nights, Randy's mom agreed to respond to the alarm and assist Randy in waking up and getting to the bathroom. Then she was to leave him on is own. If he wet his clothing and bedding, he would take off his wet clothes, lay them by the hamper, put his dry clothing and bedding on, reattach his sensor, review the steps in his mind, and go back to bed. Each morning he recorded his score on the board.

The first week was Spring Training and it took Randy sev-

eral nights to wake up and respond to the alarm. He and his mom were pretty worn out from their nighttime events. His score was Bend Bandits 6, Randy's Rockies 1. As was his assignment every week, he called his continence nurse, whom he now called Coach, and reported his score. The first week he told her of his response and how his mother helped early in the week. His first "run" or point was on the 6th night (inning) and he did feel encouragement. By weeks three and four, Randy was feeling more confident and having 2 to 4 points (or dry nights). He was still encouraged and motivated to go the distance of 10 weeks. By weeks 7 and 8 he was well on his way to winning the games each week and having few leaks. At week 10 he was ready to enter the World Series and became a champion. His reward was a trip to Coors Field with his dad to see the Rockies play.

This program was not easy for a young boy of seven. It required a great deal of motivation, effort and support. But the affect it had on Randy's confidence, his self-esteem, the family dynamics, and his enthusiasm to join his friends in overnight events was extremely positive. Perhaps Randy would have outgrown his bedwetting by 8 or 9 or 10 years of age. Most continence professionals agree that behavioral programs can speed this development and are worth a consistent effort.

Randy said, "Coach, I can do the alarm, the bathroom, the whole thing all by myself. It is not big deal. I hardly ever have to change my bed. Now my brother is jealous because I got to see the Rockies play."

Responses to behavioral therapy vary, depending on the person's symptoms and ability to do the changes. As you can see from the discussion, some will have to do several behavioral therapy options. A major benefit is the fact that the behaviors are not harmful. But they must be performed to be effective.

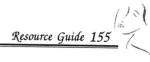

ଏ *Chapter 7* ଙ୍

Resource Guide

Organizations

Agency for Health Care Policy and Research,
(Now Agency for Healthcare Research and Quality)
Understanding Incontinence: Patient Guide
> P.O. Box 8547
> Silver Springs, MD 20907
> 800-358-9295
> www.ahcpr.gov

Bladder Health Council American Foundation for Urologic
Diseases
> 1128 N. Charles St.
> Baltimore, MD 21201
> (800) 242-2383
> www.afud.org

DesChutes Medical Products, Inc.
> 1011 SW Emkay Dr., Suite 104
> Bend, OR 97702
> (800) 323-1363
> www.deschutesmed.com

Incontinence Information Center
> P.O. Box 9
> Minneapolis, MN 55440
> (800) 843-5440
> fax: (612) 930-6654

Interstitial Cystitis Association of America
> P.O. Box 1553
> Madison Square Station
> New York, NY 10159
> (800) 422-1626
> fax: (212) 677-6139
> www.ichelp.org

National Association for Continence
P.O. Box 8310
Spartanburg, SC 29305
(800) 252-3337
fax: (864) 579-7902
www.nafc.org

National Kidney and Urologic Information Clearinghouse
3 Information Way
Bethseda, MD 20892-3580
(800) 891-5388
fax: (301) 907-8906
www.niddk.nih.gov

Simon Foundation for Continence
P.O. Box 815
Wilmette, Il 60091
(800) 237-4666
fax: (847) 864-9758
www.simonfoundation.org

The Canadian Continence Foundation
B.P./P.O. 66524
Cavendish Mall
Crote S. Luc, Quebec
Canada H4W3J6
800-265-9575
fax: 514-932-3533
www.continence-fdn.ca

The National Enuresis Society
7777 Forest Lane, Suite C-737
Dallas, TX 75230-2518
(800) 637-8080
www.peds.umn.edu/centers/nes

Professional Organizations

American College of Obstetrics and Gynecology
P.O. Box 96920
Washington, DC 20090-6920
(202) 638-5577
fax: (202) 863-4994
www.acog.org

American Physical Therapy Association
1111 North Fairfax Street
Alexandria, VA 22314-1488
(703) 684-2782
fax: (703)684-7343
www.apta.org

American Urogynecologic Society
401 N. Michigan Avenue
Chicago, IL 60611
(312) 644-6610
fax: (312) 245-1084
www.augs.org

American Urological Association, Inc.
1120 North Charles Street
Baltimore, MD 21201-5559
(410) 727-1100
fax: (410) 223-4370
www.auanet.org

American Association of Rehabilitation Nurses
4700 W. Lake Avenue
Glenview, IL 60025-1485
(847) 375-4710
fax: (847) 375-4777
www.rehabnurse.org

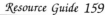

International Continence Society
The Continence Foundation
2 Doughty Street
London WCIN 2PH
44-714046875
www.continet.org.sg

National Alliance of Nurse Practitioners
325 Pennsylvania Avenue SE
Washington, DC 20003-1100
(202) 675-6350

Society of Urologic Nurses and Associates
East Holly Avenue, Box 56
Pitman, NJ 08071-00565
(609) 256-2335
fax: (609) 589-7463
www.suna.org

Wound, Ostomy, and Continence Nurses Society
1550 S. Coast Highway, Suite 201
Laguna Beach, CA 92651
(888) 224-9626
fax: (714) 376-3456
www.wocn.org

References

1 Newman JL (1962, June 30). *Old folk in wet beds.* British Medical Journal, 1824-1827.
2 Wagner TH & Hu T (1998). *Economic costs of urinary incontinence in 1995.* Urology 51(3): 355-361.
3 Appell RA (1999). *Pathophysiology of urge incontinence.* Contemporary Urology March: 1-6.
4 Sherman RA, Davis GD, Wong MF (1997). *Behavioral treatment of exercise-induced urinary incontinence among female soldiers.* Military Medicine 162: 690-694.
5 Bavendam TG & Gartley CB (1997). *The personal side of incontinence* in O'Donnell, PD (ed). *Urinary Incontinence;* St. Louis: Mosby, 1-4.
6 Ettinger WH, Mitchell BS, Blair SN. (1996) *Fitness after 50;* St. Louis: Beverly Cracom Publications.
7 Rejeski WJ, Kenney EA. (1988) Fitness motivation. Champaign, IL: Human Kinetics.
8 Nygaard IE, Thompson FL, Svengalis SL, & Albright JP. (1994) *Urinary incontinence in elite nulliparous athletes.* Obstetrics and Gynecology 84: 183-187.
9 vonEschenbach AC, Rodriguez DB. (1981) *Sexual rehabilitation of the urologic cancer patient.* Boston: GK Hall, 10.
10 Sheldon CA, Wacksman J. *Enuresis* in O'Donnell, PD (ed). (1997) *Urinary Incontinence;* St. Louis: Mosby; 163-170.

Glossary

Alzheimer disease: A type of dementia, characterized by confusion, memory loss, disorientation.

Bedwetter: Incontinent of urine at night while in bed.

Biofeedback: A process providing a person information about her body through the use of instrumentation, such as blood pressure or muscle contraction.

Bladder: The muscular sac in the pelvis that stores urine.

Bladder control: Ability to voluntarily keep urine from leaking out of the bladder.

Bladder drill: (see bladder training) A system of therapy for incontinence in which a patient practices holding urine for increasing increments of time.

Bladder suspension: A surgical procedure to position the bladder and prevent descention in to the vagina.

Bladder training: Another term for bladder drill, a system of therapy for incontinence in which a patient practices holding urine for increasing increments of time.

Burch procedure: A surgical procedure for stress incontinence, the urethra is stabilized to prevent mobility and leakage.

Chronic incontinence: Urinary leakage that has occurred for over 6 months and not of a temporary nature.

Congestive heart failure: A condition where the heart as a pump cannot perform its functions good enough to keep blood circulating throughout the body.

Constipation: Difficulty in passing stool or passing of hard stools.

Cystocele: Protrusion or hernia of the bladder in to the vagina.

Diabetes: A clinical condition where there is a decrease or lack of insulin secretion to metabolize sugars, characterized by increase in urine output.

Diuretic medication: A drug that promotes the excretion of urine.

Double void: A technique for emptying the bladder, essentially trying to empty the bladder twice in a short space of time.

Elasticity: Ability of tissue to regain its original shape after stretching.

Electrical stimulation: A process where electrodes, either implanted or on the surface of the body, convey a small electrical current for therapeutic purposes.

Estrogen: The female hormone, responsible for secondary sex characteristics of the female, important in vaginal, urethral and pelvic muscle strength.

Rectocele: A protrusion or hernia of the rectum in to the vagina.

Rectum: The portion of the colon just above the anus, or outside opening.

Reflex incontinence: Loss of bladder control related to a problem in the spinal cord.

Self-dehydration: Limiting fluid intake, enough to cause dehydration or excessive loss of water from the body.

Skin breakdown: A break in the skin integrity, an ulcer or abrasion.

Sleepwetting (see bedwetter): Incontinent of urine while asleep.

Sphincter: A circular band of muscle fibers that can close a natural opening in the bladder, a valve, like the bladder sphincters.

Stress incontinence: Loss of urine related to physical exertion, usually associated with pelvic floor weakness or sphincter insufficiency.

Transient incontinence: Loss of bladder control that is temporary, such as related to a urinary tract infection (treat the infection and the incontinence is resolved).

Ureters: Two tubes connecting the kidneys to the bladder.

Urethra: Tube connecting the bladder to the outside of the body.

Urge incontinence: Loss of bladder control characterized by frequent and urgent need to go to the bathroom.

Urinary tract infection: Infection of the kidneys or bladder.

Uterus: Female organ of reproduction, lies behind and just above the bladder.

Vagina: Female canal to the uterus, lies behind the bladder and in front of the rectum.

Vaginal weights: Cones designed to be used by females when strengthening the pelvic muscles to treat incontinence.

Voiding: The act of urinating, to empty the bladder.

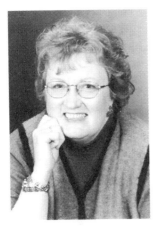

About the Author

Dorothy B. Smith is a nurse who has worked with incontinence patients in acute care and long-term care settings, assisted living, clinics, and home care. She is the author of over 125 professional publications related to her field and has given numerous presentations in the US, Canada, and Europe. She has been editor of The Journal of Wound, Ostomy and Continence Nursing and Dimensions in Oncology Nursing. Ms. Smith has received nursing and publication honors from The University of Texas M.D. Anderson Cancer Center (Brown Award), The Oncology Nursing Society (Mara Mogensen Flaherty Award), the Wound, Ostomy and Continence Nurses Society (manuscript award), The Texas Medical Center (essay award), The American Medical Writers Association (book award) and is a Fellow in The American Academy of Nursing. She is certified by the Wound, Ostomy and Continence Nursing Society. Currently she is Vice President, Clinical Affairs for DesChutes Medical Products, Inc., Bend, Oregon, a research and development company for pelvic floor dysfunction. Dorothy is married and has one daughter.